CARDIOLOGY REVISION

For

David and Andrew

CARDIOLOGY REVISION
CASE HISTORIES, MCQs AND DATA INTERPRETATION

ALISTAIR MACKAY BSc MD MRCP
Senior Registrar in Medicine
Edinburgh Royal Infirmary

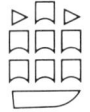

CHURCHILL LIVINGSTONE
EDINBURGH LONDON MELBOURNE AND NEW YORK 1985

CHURCHILL LIVINGSTONE
Medical Division of Longman Group Limited

Distributed in the United States of America by Churchill Livingstone Inc., 1560 Broadway, New York, N.Y. 10036, and by associated companies, branches and representatives throughout the world.

© Longman Group Limited, 1985

All rights reserved. No part of this publication may be reproduced, stored in a retrieval system, or transmitted in any form or by any means, electronic, mechanical, photocopying, recording or otherwise, without the prior permission of the publishers (Churchill Livingstone, Robert Stevenson House, 1-3 Baxter's Place, Leith Walk, Edinburgh EH1 3AF).

First published 1985

ISBN 0443 02748 X

British Library Cataloging in Publication Data
Mackay, Alistair
  Cardiology revision
  1. Cardiology
  I. Title
  616.1'2   RC681

Library of Congress Cataloguing in Publication Data Mackay, Alistair.
  Cardiology revision.

  Includes index.
  1. Heart—Diseases—Case studies. 2. Cardiology—Examinations, questions, etc. I. Title. [DNLM: 1. Cardiology—Examination questions. WG 18 M153c]
  RC682.M25   1984   616.1'209   83-15210

Printed in Singapore by Selector Printing Co (Pte) Ltd

PREFACE

Cardiology revision is designed to assist candidates preparing to sit Parts I and II of the MRCP (or equivalent) examinations. Although it touches on most topics pertaining to cardiology and hypertension, it does not claim to be a comprehensive cardiology text: a suggested reading list is appended.

The book contains three sections. In the first 'grey' cases are supplemented by multiple choice questions apposite to subjects raised in each case. In the second, readers are asked to interpret radiographic, electrocardiographic, cardiac catheter, biochemical and haematological data, including electrocardiogram recordings from patients with implanted pacemakers: since M-mode echocardiography is now a widely available technique a small number of echocardiograms is also included for interpretation. In the third section is a series of linked multiple choice questions, set at various points as the presentation, investigation and subsequent management of a number of patients is unfolded. All case histories and data are based on patients in whose management the author has been involved in the Western Infirmary, Glasgow, and the Royal Infirmary, Edinburgh. Explanatory notes amplify answers to each question. A subject index is included.

Thanks are due to Dr David de Bono for his encouragement in the preparation of this book, to Ian Ramsden for his expertise in the preparation of the illustrations and to Lesley Cook for secretarial help. Those who have not attempted to write a thesis or textbook will not appreciate the inroads which such an exercise makes on the writer's time. Particular thanks are therefore due to my wife and family for their patience and understanding during the writing of this book.

Edinburgh, 1985   A.M.

CONTENTS

SECTION 1

Grey cases: Case histories followed by questions   1
and MCQ

SECTION 2

Interpretation
  X-rays   164
  Electrocardiograms   184
  Data   207
  Picture quiz   216
  Echocardiograms   221

SECTION 3

Linked cases: Case histories interspersed with   225
relevant MCQ questions
Further reading   253
Index   254

1
GREY CASES

PATIENT 1

Answers are on pages 5–7

HISTORY

An 18 year old labourer is referred from a peripheral hospital for further management because of cardiomegaly, persisting tachycardia and weight loss of 4 kg. The patient was well until 4 weeks previously when he developed nausea, malaise, upper abdominal and chest discomfort which worsened on inspiration and movement, and dyspnoea precipitated by progressively less exertion. He smokes 15 cigarettes per day, and drinks up to 4 pints of beer each night. Two sibs and both parents are in good health.

EXAMINATION

BP 110/80 mmHg. Pulse — 110 beats per minute, regular, small volume. Apex beat displaced to the sixth intercostal space in the anterior axillary line. S3 present. Intermittent midsystolic murmur at the apex. 2 cm smooth non-tender hepatomegaly. No splenomegaly.

QUESTIONS

1. What is the differential diagnosis?

2. Apart from the chest X–ray and ECG what investigations do you think are important?

3. What are the most important aspects of management of this patient?

Multiple choice questions

4. A third heart sound:

- T (a) *may be normal in young people*
- T (b) *is a common finding in patients with thyrotoxicosis*
- F (c) *is situated in late diastole*
- F (d) *is of high frequency*
- T (e) *is a characteristic finding in patients with pericardial constriction*

5. Alcohol may affect the heart by:

- T (a) *protecting against coronary artery disease in modest doses*
- F (b) *producing high output cardiac failure due to riboflavine deficiency*
- T (c) *precipitating sudden death*
- T (d) *producing atrial fibrillation as part of a generalized cardiomyopathy*
- F (e) *stimulating muscle growth*

6. An intermittent apical systolic murmur:

- F (a) *is a characteristic finding in hypertrophic cardiomyopathy*
- T (b) *may be caused by dilatation of the mitral valve ring*
- T (c) *may be an innocent finding in teenagers*
- F F (d) *is common in atrial septal defect*
- T T (e) *may be suggestive of subacute bacterial endocarditis*

7. In Bornholm disease:

- F (a) *relapse is rare after chest pain has remitted*
- T (b) *opiate is often required to control chest pain*

F (c) *no ECG changes occur*

F (d) *tetracycline is the treatment of choice*

F (e) *most cases occur in the late autumn/early winter*

8. Which of the following conditions are recognized causes of cardiomyopathy?

T (a) *Glycogen storage disease*

T (b) *Diphtheria*

T (c) *Malaria*

F (d) *Diabetes insipidus*

T (e) *Hereditary spherocytosis*

ANSWERS AND DISCUSSION

PATIENT 1

1. The differential diagnosis in a young man without significant valvular disease or hypertension and in the presence of cardiomegaly and a low output state is that of congestive cardiomyopathy, be this infective (particularly viral) myopericarditis, the result of alcohol, of toxic agents such as cobalt or some antimitotic drugs, or of metabolic disorders, or idiopathic in nature. In view of the prodromal symptoms the likeliest explanation would be viral myopericarditis.

2. Investigations — to be undertaken would be:

— full blood count, differential white count, and ESR
— for evidence of autoimmune disorders such as A.N.F.
— viral antibody titres
— liver enzymes

— non invasive tests to assess left ventricular function and/or confirm absence of valvular disease, i.e. echocardiography, radionuclide ventriculography
— invasive tests — cardiac catheterization, ventriculography and coronary angiography
— cardiac biopsy
These invasive tests should be reserved until non invasive means have failed to establish the diagnosis

3. Bed rest.

Treat cardiac failure with diuretics, plus unload the heart with vasodilators/venodilators as appropriate. Treat arrhythmias as they arise.

Be aware of the possible need for anticoagulants — there is a high incidence of systemic and pulmonary emboli.

Valve replacement may be relevant as may consideration of cardiac transplantation in a few severe selected cases.

4. TRUE   TRUE   FALSE   FALSE   TRUE

The third heart sound is a low frequency sound, associated with rapid left ventricular filling as in young people or thyrotoxic patients, or in patients with a high filling pressure secondary to myocardial disease. The speedy termination of diastolic ventricular filling in patients with pericardial constriction also results in a sharp S3 or pericardial 'knock'.

5. TRUE   FALSE   TRUE   TRUE   FALSE

Whether alcohol in modest amounts protects against coronary artery disease is a matter of debate with the balance of evidence at present in favour of such an effect. The toxic effects are much better documented with a picture of congestive cardiomyopathy as a result of direct toxic effects and/or thiamine, not riboflavine, deficiency. Atrial fibrillation is a characteristic finding in this cardiomyopathy but often reverts to sinus rhythm with abstention. Sudden death, probably due to ventricular fibrillation, is not uncommon in young alcoholics.

6. FALSE   TRUE   TRUE   FALSE   TRUE

The systolic murmur of hypertrophic cardiomyopathy is generated partly by left ventricular outflow tract obstruction and partly by mitral regurgitation which is usually present to some degree — characteristically the murmurs once present are a constant feature though a variety of manoeuvres, physiological and pharmacological, may vary the intensity of the murmurs. Intermittent mild mitral regurgitation secondary to dilatation of the left heart including the mitral ring is common in much myocardial disease. In teenagers the innocent systolic murmurs usually arise from the pulmonary outflow tract but may be heard at the apex also. The systolic murmur in atrial septal defect arises from the pulmonary valve. Variable murmurs are a well known accompaniment of S.B.E.

7. FALSE   TRUE   FALSE   FALSE   FALSE

Bornholm disease or epidemic myalgia is caused by Coxsackie B 1-5 viruses (Coxsackie B 2-5 may cause myopericarditis). ECG abnormalities of myopericardial involvement therefore often accompany the myalgia. Epidemics usually occur in the summer. Symptomatic treatment is all that is available, relapses are not uncommon, and the pain (devil's grip) may be so severe that opiate is required for a period to control this.

8. TRUE   TRUE   TRUE   FALSE   FALSE

Glycogen may be deposited in cardiac muscle cells, especially in Pompe disease. One of the most serious consequences of diphtheria is the myocarditic effects of diphtheria toxin. Plasmodium falciparum malaria is often accompanied by myocardial involvement which may be apparent on the ECG, though the effects of the protozoa on other organs may overshadow the cardiac complications. Diabetes insipidus and hereditary spherocytosis are not associated with cardiomyopathy.

PATIENT 2

Answers are on pages 10–12

HISTORY

A 27 year old joiner presents with a 3 week history of persistent cough, purulent brown spit, intermittent fever, and sharp chest pain variable in its site and intensity, but exacerbated by coughing and movement. He is on no regular medication and his only previous hospital admission was as a child when he experienced encephalitis complicating chickenpox. He lives with his girlfriend and has no children. His parents and family are all in good health. He smokes 20 cigarettes per day and admits to drinking 2 pints of lager on most nights.

EXAMINATION

On examination he appears flushed (38.3°C) and his sclerae are mildly icteric. He has no palmar erythema or spider naevi but has many scratch marks on his arms. His liver is palpable 6 cm below the right costal margin in the mid clavicular line but the spleen is not palpable. BP 140/80 mmHg. Pulse — 100 beats per minute, regular, normal character. A soft poorly conducted systolic murmur is audible at the apex and left sternal edge. At the base of the right lung there is a pleural rub.

ECG shows sinus tachycardia.
Chest X-ray shows linear atelectasis in the left mid-zone.

QUESTIONS

1. What are the likely diagnoses?

2. What four investigations do you think are most important?

3. What treatment is likely to be of benefit?

Multiple choice questions

4. Symptoms frequently present in subacute bacterial endocarditis include:

(a) *lumbar backache*

(b) *dysphagia*

(c) *weight loss*

(d) *hoarseness*

(e) *dyspnoea*

5. Antibiotic cover should be advocated for the following procedures in patients with mitral stenosis:

(a) *urethral dilatation*

(b) *liver biopsy*

(c) *dental scaling*

(d) *barium enema*

(e) *fibreoptic bronchoscopy*

6. Antibiotic cover for dental extractions should be advocated in the following conditions:

(a) *coarctation of the aorta*

(b) *hypertrophic cardiomyopathy*

(c) *ventricular septal defect*

(d) *aortic sclerosis*

(e) *Bjork-Shiley mitral prosthesis.*

7. Which of the following statements is/are true concerning subacute bacterial endocarditis.

F (a) The incidence of SBE has undergone a steady fall since the 1940s.

T (b) Endocarditis within the atria is unusual in atrial septal defect.

T (c) Anaemia is always present in SBE.

T (d) Cardiac failure resulting from acute aortic regurgitation is the commonest cause of death in bacterial endocarditis.

T (e) Emboli occluding the arteries to the legs are commoner with fungal infection of the aortic and mitral valves.

8. The diagnosis of subacute bacterial endocarditis:

F (a) is excluded by six negative blood cultures

T (b) is confirmed by a single positive blood culture

F (c) should not be suspected unless a changing murmur is heard

F (d) is excluded in a persistently apyrexial patient

T (e) is supported by the presence of hypergammaglobulinaemia.

ANSWERS AND DISCUSSION

PATIENT 2

1. A crucial observation in this case is the presence of 'scratch' marks only on the arms of a jaundiced patient — this raises the strong suspicion of drug abuse. Likely diagnoses are thus viral hepatitis, and recurrent pulmonary emboli. Given the suspicion of drug abuse infective endocarditis of structures on the right side of the heart with infective emboli is likely. If endocarditis of the right side of the heart is severe producing right heart failure, jaundice may result from this.

2. Blood cultures
   Echocardiography
   Viral screen, including hepatitis B surface antigen
   Liver function tests

3. Appropriate antibiotic or antifungal drugs may cure the endocarditis. If profound right heart failure occurs secondary to a regurgitant tricuspid valve, valve replacement may be indicated. Symptomatic measures may be helpful in the management of viral hepatitis.

4. TRUE   FALSE   TRUE   FALSE   TRUE

5. TRUE   TRUE   TRUE   TRUE   FALSE

6. TRUE   TRUE   TRUE   TRUE   TRUE

7. FALSE TRUE   TRUE   TRUE   TRUE

8. FALSE FALSE   FALSE FALSE   TRUE

Subacute bacterial endocarditis may produce symptoms affecting most systems in the body and thus may mimic many diseases ranging from tuberculosis to carcinoma of the stomach. Among these symptoms dyspnoea and weight loss are common, while persistent lumbar ache apparently unrelated to renal or vertebral involvement by emboli is an increasingly recognized early complaint. Dysphagia and hoarseness are not usually related to SBE.

Unequivocal evidence of the benefits of chemoprophylaxis in situations of transient bacteraemia is lacking, but most clinicians would recommend such prophylaxis. Instrumentation of the urogenital tract, dental scaling and liver biopsy constitute such situations, though fibreoptic, in contrast to rigid, bronchoscopy is not usually associated with bacteraemia.

Again statistical proof of the value of chemoprophylaxis in much cardiac disease is lacking. However where there is or has been distortion of any structure in the heart or great vessels, even if this has been corrected surgically, and particularly if foreign material has been implanted, it is current practice to employ prophylactic antibiotics at the time of surgical procedures. This should also apply to the abnormal valve in aortic sclerosis.

Over the past 20 years the decline in the incidence of SBE has levelled out and the trend has reversed. Where there is a small pressure gradient as in atrial septal defect, SBE is unusual. Anaemia is generally thought to be a uniform feature of the condition. Acute left heart failure as a result of destruction of the aortic valve is the commonest cause of death in bacterial endocarditis. Fungal infection of the valves produces larger thrombi which usually lodge in major vessels in the pelvis or legs.

Negative cultures by no means exclude SBE — indeed culture-negative SBE forms a distinct subgroup of the condition. A single positive culture may be a helpful result but may merely be due to a contaminant. No murmur need be heard in SBE, and particularly in older patients a temperature persistently within the accepted normal range may be found. Elevated serum globulins are often found, and it is thought that antigen-antibody reactions or deposition of circulating immune complexes are responsible for many of the clinical manifestations of the disease in kidneys, joints, and skin including splinter haemorrhages and Osler nodes.

PATIENT 3

Answers are on pages 15–18

HISTORY

A 28 year old architect is noted during an insurance examination to have a blood pressure of 180/105 mmHg, and is referred to the medical outpatient clinic. He is asymptomatic, a non smoker, with no family history of vascular disease, and is surprised at the fuss being made.

QUESTIONS

1. What physical signs would you be interested in looking for?

2. How would you manage this patient?

3. Are investigations indicated, and if so what?

Multiple choice questions

4. When an abdominal bruit is discovered in a hypertensive patient:

(a) *essential hypertension is the likeliest diagnosis*

(b) *the finding is pathognomonic of renal artery stenosis*

(c) *it signifies a very tight stenosis of the renal artery*

14 CARDIOLOGY REVISION

(d) it is a good prognostic sign if renal artery surgery is contemplated

(e) auscultation over the back may be helpful in lateralising the abnormality.

5. In patients with essential hypertension:

(a) dietary salt intake is commonly greater than in age-and sex-matched normotensive patients from the same population

(b) an excess of sodium is commonly found in blood cells

(c) mean exchangeable sodium is not significantly different from that in age and sex matched controls

(d) microscopic evidence of adrenal hyperplasia is not an unusual finding

(e) dietary salt restriction may return blood pressure to normal.

6. In the measurement of blood pressure:

(a) the use of a standard 14 cm cuff in an obese patient will lead to an underestimate of the true blood pressure

(b) mean arterial pressure equals the diastolic value plus one quarter of the difference between systolic and diastolic values

(c) a single casual blood pressure reading in a general practitioner's surgery has little relevance to long term morbidity and mortality

(d) admission to hospital for 24 hours commonly precipitates a slight but significant rise in blood pressure

(e) 'Normal' blood pressure varies with age.

7. Blood pressure may be raised acutely by:

(a) performing mental arithmetic

(b) smoking a cigarette

(c) abdominal palpation in a patient with an adrenal cortical tumour

(d) *driving a car*

(e) *parenteral ergotamine in migraine management.*

8. The following are indicative of left ventricular hypertrophy on an electrocardiogram:

(a) $S_{V1} + R_{V6} = 40$ *mm in an 18 year old negro*

(b) *R in aVL* $= 18$ *mm in a 40 year old woman*

(c) *R in* $V_6 = 22$ *mm with plane ST depression of 1 mm and deep T wave inversion in a 60 year old man*

(d) *R in* $V_5 = 35$ *mm in a 46 year old woman*

(e) *R in aVF* $= 20$ *mm in an 80 year old woman*

ANSWERS AND DISCUSSION

PATIENT 3

1. Physical signs

(a) Blood pressure in both arms after lying for 10 minutes and standing for two minutes. Optic fundal examination. Position and character of the apex beat. Evidence of left ventricular failure.

(b) Related to a cause for the hypertension: delay in the femoral pulses. Abdominal bruit. Abdominal masses. Stigmata of Cushing's syndrome or collagenosis. Subtle or overt signs of alcohol excess since elevation of blood pressure may occur during alcohol withdrawal.

2. The patient should be reviewed several times with multiple BP recordings so that the effects of temporary sympathetic stimulation will be minimized. Full explanation about the significance of BP elevation in relation to longterm morbidity and mortality and with respect to further investigation should be given. Development of rapport between physician and patient will contribute to good longterm compliance should treatment prove necessary. Thiazide diuretics or beta adrenergic neurone blockers would be the agent of first choice in this patient.

3. Investigation is indicated. A BP of 180/105 mmHg is undoubtedly high for a 28 year old man. The following tests would be useful: full blood count, serum urea, creatinine and electrolyte concentrations; creatinine clearance; 24 hour urinary normetadrenaline level; intravenous urography; isotope renography. Some authorities would make a good case for renal arteriography being performed in a patient such as this even in the absence of clear urographic abnormalities. Estimation of plasma renin angiotensin II and aldosterone concentrations under baseline conditions of diet and posture, the patient having received no medication for 3-4 weeks, may be helpful. Also baseline chest X-ray and ECG.

4. TRUE FALSE FALSE FALSE TRUE

The absence of an abdominal bruit may indicate no renal artery stenosis, mild stenosis, severe stenosis or total occulsion. If a bruit is present it may indicate 65-85% narrowing of the renal artery, but since a bruit may arise from an atheromatous aorta in a patient with essential hypertension and essential hypertension is a much commoner diagnosis in the hypertensive population than renal artery stenosis, an abdominal bruit is an unreliable physical sign as far as the diagnosis of renal artery stenosis is concerned. It has no prognostic value. Auscultation over the back may help to lateralize the abnormal renal artery if such is the source of the bruit.

5. FALSE TRUE TRUE TRUE TRUE

The relationship between the level of salt in the diet and the prevalence, or indeed the aetiology, of essential hypertension has been, and still is, the subject of much debate. A cause and effect relationship is far from proven though excess sodium in red and white blood cells has been documented. Mean exchangeable sodium is not different in patients with essential hypertension compared with age and sex matched controls, though a positive and significant statistical correlation between total exchangeable sodium and arterial pressure has been identified. Salt restriction was an early and successful if unpalatable means of lowering blood pressure (e.g. 'Kempener rice diet') and in moderation is still a useful adjunct to therapy. Micronodular hyperplasia of the adrenal glands is a relatively frequent finding in essential hypertension, and does not reflect a form of primary hyperaldosteronism as previously thought.

6. FALSE   FALSE   FALSE   FALSE   TRUE

An inappropriately small cuff (the inflatable part of the cuff being less than two thirds of the circumference of the arm) will produce an overestimate of blood pressure, and vice versa. Mean arterial pressure equals the diastolic value (fifth Korotkof sound) plus one third of the pulse pressure. The Framingham study among others has shown that even one casual blood pressure recording correlates well with long-term morbidity and mortality. A gradual fall in blood pressure over the first 24 or 48 hours is a common finding in newly admitted patients. 'Normal' blood pressure is difficult to define but there is persuasive and valid epidemiological evidence that it rises with age.

7. TRUE   TRUE   FALSE   TRUE   TRUE

Through liberation of sympathetic amines any form of harrassment such as driving a car or performing mental arithmetic may raise blood pressure temporarily. Through release of adrenal catecholamines and by actions on the central nervous system and on autonomic ganglia nicotine may acutely raise blood pressure. Parenteral or indeed intranasal ergotamine may directly raise blood pressure by its own action on arterial walls. Abdominal palpation may provoke a hypertensive crisis in a patient with a phaeochromocytoma not an adrenal cortical adenoma.

8. FALSE TRUE FALSE TRUE TRUE

Accepted criteria for diagnosing left ventricular hypertrophy from the standard 12 lead electrocardiogram vary from centre to centre. The current criteria recommended by the World Health Organisation expert committee (1980) are based on the longstanding Sokolow–Lyon index – $S_{V1} + R_{V6}$ greater than 35 mm. However in young people and those with thin chest walls a measurement of up to 40 mm would be accepted by most as being within normal limits. An isolated chest lead finding of an R or S wave in excess of 30 mm would be accepted as evidence of hypertrophy; so also would an R or S wave in excess of 20 mm (some would accept 18 mm) in a limb lead be accepted as evidence of hypertrophy. Plane ST depression with repolarization changes is indicative of myocardial ischaemia; taken together with an R wave in V6 of 22 mm, they still do not constitute evidence of left ventricular hypertrophy and 'strain', though a deep S wave in lead V1 in the same patient would provide sufficient additional evidence.

PATIENT 4

Answers are on pages 21–23

HISTORY

A 50 year old housewife is admitted to hospital following severe retrosternal discomfort of rapid onset with nausea, vomiting, dyspnoea and collapse. She gives no past history of chest pain, but 2 weeks previously she experienced severe 'heartburn' for 2 hours though this resolved spontaneously and she did not seek medical help. Her only other history is of moderate hypertension for 10 years, treated with methyldopa. She smokes 15 cigarettes per day.

EXAMINATION

On examination the patient is pale, sweating and obese. BP 170/90 mmHg in the right arm lying. Sinus tachycardia 110 per minute. Apex beat in 5th inter-costal space in the anterior axillary line. Loud midsystolic murmur over the whole precardium with a loud descrendo diastolic murmur at the left sternal edge particularly. Bilateral basal crepitations present.

ECG: Sinus tachycardia. S V_1 + R V_6 = 46 mm. T wave inversion in aVL and $V_4 - V_6$.

QUESTIONS

1. What is the differential diagnosis?

2. What other aspects of physical examination may be helpful?

3. Which investigations are required?

4. How would you manage this patient?

5. 24 hours later the patient is found to be anuric. What explanations are likely?

Multiple choice questions

6. The severity of aortic regurgitation may be gauged by:
   (a) the intensity of the murmur
   (b) the harshness of the murmur
   (c) the duration of the murmur
   (d) the situation of maximum intensity of the murmur
   (e) the loudness of the accompanying systolic murmur.

7. Marfan's syndrome:
   (a) is inherited as a Mendelian autosomal dominant trait
   (b) is associated with an increased incidence of SBE of the mitral valve
   (c) often includes retinal detachment
   (d) is very rarely the result of a mutation
   (e) is usually associated with dilatation of the aorta and great vessels but rarely of the heart itself.

8. Mitral valve prolapse:
   (a) occurs in the majority of patients with Marfan's syndrome
   (b) is associated with a high incidence of sudden death
   (c) is exacerbated by the Valsalva manoeuvre
   (d) is often accompanied by T wave changes in the inferior leads of the ECG

(e) *often leads to amaurosis fugax.*

9. Factors predisposing to dissection of the aorta include:

(a) *pregnancy*

(b) *pseudoxanthoma elasticum*

(c) *trauma*

(d) *portal hypertension*

(e) *systemic hypertension*

10. Which of the following statements is/are true?

(a) *Rheumatic valve disease is now an uncommon cause of chronic aortic regurgitation*

(b) *Exertional syncope is common in aortic regurgitation*

(c) *Use of glyceryl trinitrate is contraindicated in aortic regurgitation*

(d) *Horner's syndrome may result from aortic dissection*

(e) *ECG changes of acute myocardial infarction during aortic dissection imply a coincidental event.*

ANSWERS AND DISCUSSION

PATIENT 4

1. The findings are compatible, particularly in view of the history of hypertension, with acute aortic regurgitation due to disease of the aortic valve itself or after dissection of the aorta. The relatively minor ECG abnormalities and the severity of the collapse belie the diagnosis of myocardial infarction

in a patient with incidental aortic valve disease, though this must be included in the differential diagnosis. Oesophageal rupture is an unlikely alternative diagnosis.

2. Presence of peripheral pulses in neck, arms and legs, together with blood pressure in all four limbs. Bruits over the back, abdomen, carotid and femoral arteries may also be helpful signs. Evidence of Marfan's syndrome should be sought — unlikely in an obese woman though formes frustre exist.

3. Chest X–ray
Echocardiogram
Aortography

4. Controlled hypotension prior to emergency surgery to repair the aortic dissection is indicated.

5. Acute renal failure due to prolonged hypotension (abdominal aortic pressures may have been much lower than those in the right arm) or acute ischaemia of the kidneys, the dissection having extended to occlude the origins of the renal arteries.

6. FALSE   FALSE   TRUE   FALSE   FALSE

The severity of aortic regurgitation correlates best with the duration of the murmur. In mild regurgitation the murmur is heard in early diastole and is often high pitched. In severe regurgitation the murmur extends throughout diastole with a decrescendo pattern. Where left ventricular decompensation supervenes the late diastolic component of the murmur may be lost.

7. TRUE   TRUE   TRUE   FALSE   FALSE

Marfan's syndrome is inherited as an autosomal dominant trait with variable phenotypic expression, but may be the result of a mutation in up to 15% of patients, particularly if the parents are old. It is a generalized disorder of connective tissue affecting the heart (including the mitral valve — the commonest associated cardiac abnormality — with an increased incidence of SBE) and eye (affecting both lenticular attachments and retina) as well as great vessels, joints and bones.

8. TRUE   FALSE   TRUE   TRUE   FALSE

By echocardiography mitral valve prolapse has been shown in around 90% of patients with Marfan's syndrome. Sudden death certainly occurs in mitral valve prolapse but is not common. During the Valsalva manoeuvre cardiac size decreases, the murmur of mitral prolapse begins sooner and the intensity is often increased. Where the syndrome is associated with symptoms non specific inferior ECG changes are common. Embolic phenomena do occur with mitral valve prolapse but the incidence of amaurosis fugax is not high.

9. TRUE   TRUE   TRUE   FALSE   TRUE

Medial degeneration of the aorta appears to be a prerequisite for development of aortic dissection. Systemic hypertension and disorders of collagen formation are contributory to this process. There is a strong but ill understood association between dissection and the third trimester of pregnancy in particular. Trauma may rarely initiate dissection, but more commonly causes a localized aortic tear.

10. FALSE   FALSE   FALSE   TRUE   FALSE

Rheumatic aortic regurgitation is still a common problem. When chronic regurgitation becomes symptomatic dyspnoea, exertional and nocturnal, is common but syncope rare. Where angina occurs in aortic regurgitation nitrates may be helpful.

In aortic dissection pressure on the superior cervical sympathetic ganglion may produce Horner's syndrome. Concurrent myocardial infarction probably implies dissection of the aorta back to involve the orifice of a coronary artery.

PATIENT 5

Answers are on pages 27–29

HISTORY

A 66 year old retired teacher presents to the accident and emergency department with nausea and retching which have been unremitting for 2 hours. He has a past history of cholelithiasis but is adamant that his present problems are totally different from any previous biliary symptoms. He claims to be teetotal and has never smoked. His only other complaint is of hesitancy of micturition.

EXAMINATION

On examination he is restless, pale and in distress. BP 120/65 mmHg in the left arm, lying. Pulse regular, 50 beats per minute. Heart sounds pure. No murmurs. No crepitations. Abdomen — diffuse upper abdominal tenderness, but no rebound tenderness; bowel sounds normal; no organomegaly.
    Chest X-ray normal.
    Supine abdominal X-ray — normal gas shadows, no calcified gallstones.
    ECG shows sinus bradycardia 50/minute, but is otherwise normal.

QUESTIONS

1. What is the differential diagnosis?

2. What investigations would you perform urgently?

6 weeks later after discharge from hospital the patient complains of intermittent swelling of his left hand, and upper arm discomfort on brushing his hair.

3. What is the likely diagnosis?

4. What treatment would you offer?

Multiple choice questions

5. Following myocardial infarction:

(a) *elective surgery should be delayed for at least one year*

(b) *a persistently elevated ESR suggests arteritis has been the likely cause of the infarct*

(c) *if complicated by complete heart block, temporary pacing should be continued for at least 2 weeks before permanent pacemaker insertion is contemplated*

(d) *complaints of persistent palpitation in the presence of a normal 24 hour ambulatory ECG recording should be treated with diazepam*

(e) *many patients experience relief from longstanding angina pectoris.*

6. Following acute mycardial infarction:

(a) *sexual intercourse should be avoided for 1 month*

(b) *heavy manual workers (e.g. miners) must be expected to give up their work*

(c) *advice on diet is important for all patients*

(d) *an exercise test is a prerequisite before entry into a rehabilitation programme*

(e) there is evidence that beta blockade started as prophylaxis against subsequent sudden death should be continued indefinitely.

7. Following a myocardial infarction:

(a) there is no legal obligation to stop driving a private car
(b) a public services vehicle licence should be surrendered but reapplication can be made after freedom from symptoms for 1 year
(c) a pilot's licence is automatically rescinded
(d) a train driver may return to work after 3 months
(e) it is the clinician's responsibility to advise heavy goods vehicle licence holders to contact the vehicle licencing centre.

8. The sinoatrial node:

(a) may be infiltrated with bile salts in obstructive jaundice such that bradycardia ensues
(b) is rarely supplied by branches of the left circumflex coronary artery
(c) is situated at the anterolateral margin of the junction between the superior vena cava and right atrium
(d) is under the influence of vagal and sympathetic nerve fibres
(e) generates and transmits impulses in such a way that both atria contract synchronously.

9. Which of the following statements are correct?

(a) Nausea following myocardial infarction may often be corrected with atropine
(b) A heavy meal may be associated with ECG changes in a patient with normal coronary arteries
(c) Diverticular disease may be associated with repolarization changes on the ECG
(d) Duodenal ulcer may mimic myocardial infarction not only symptomatically but on ECG also
(e) Nausea after digoxin is invariably a central effect of the drug.

ANSWERS AND DISCUSSION

PATIENT 5

1. Myocardial infarction — the site of the chest pain is atypical but sinus bradycardia strongly suggests inferior ischaemia or infarction.
   Pancreatitis — nausea and retching, upper abdominal discomfort and a past history of gallstones suggest pancreatitiis, but the bradycardia is against this.
   Gallstones — despite the patient's protestations the pain may be due to biliary colic, with bradycardia the vagal response to lodgement of a gallstone in the biliary tract.
   Perforation of a viscus is unlikely in the presence of normal bowel sounds and bradycardia.

2. Serum amylase, urea and electrolytes, and cardiac enzymes.

3. Shoulder-hand syndrome, or reflex neurovascular dystrophy, is an ill understood late sequel of myocardial infarction. The syndrome has other causes such as cervical disc disease, trauma, or hemiparesis, though often no cause can be identified. Characteristic features are pain, reflex vasomotor disturbance, swelling, tenderness, and osteoporosis if disuse of the limb is prolonged. It has been postulated that afferent pain fibres initiate a series of reflexes through internuncial neurones with efferent autonomic and motor impulses. The symptoms/signs may begin weeks or months after the causative insult, and may last for 3-6 months. If the syndrome is severe and prolonged, atrophy and contractures may occur.

4. Physiotherapy and salicylates, or non-steroidal anti-inflammatory agents such as indomethacin, are the mainstay of treatment. Occasionally local or systemic steroids may be helpful.

5. FALSE FALSE TRUE TRUE TRUE

Elective surgery is usually delayed for 3 months after myocardial infarction, thouugh the figure is arbitrary. An elevated ESR is more suggestive of Dressler's syndrome, or the post-myocardial infarction syndrome, than of arteritis which is a rare cause of infarction. Most heart block returns to normal rhythm after myocardial infarction — permanent pacing should be delayed because of this, because of the potentially arrhythmogenic nature of the procedure, and to allow scar formation to commence in the infarct area — penetration of the myocardium with the electrode (especially of the helifix type) is not unknown. Cardiac neurosis (da Costa's syndrome) is a relatively common sequel to myocardial infarction, and may be an intractable problem. If there is significant coronary artery disease in one vessel only then infarction may indeed lead to relief from angina pectoris.

6. TRUE FALSE TRUE TRUE FALSE

Sudden vigorous exercise should be discouraged in the early weeks after myocardial infarction, but physical activity in the long term must be tailored to the individual's capabilities. An exercise tolerance test under controlled conditions in patients who may have severe disease over and above that affecting the infarcted area is a prerequisite for a medically supervised rehabilitation scheme. Obesity should be discouraged in patients with coronary artery disease, though the importance of specific advice on diets rich in polyunsaturated fats is unclear unless patients have overt hyperlipidaemia. The outcome of withdrawal of prophylactic beta blockade after one year in post-infarction patients is as yet unknown.

7. TRUE FALSE TRUE FALSE TRUE

Holders of licences, be they ordinary, HGV or PSV, are required by law to inform their licensing centre of the change in their circumstances; the clinician's duty is to advise the patient of his responsibility. Holders of an ordinary licence are advised not to drive during the first 2 months after a myocardial infarction, or if angina pectoris is easily provoked during driving thereafter. Former licencees will not be permitted to hold HGV or PSV licences after a myocardial infarction, nor will pilots. Train drivers are not permitted to be in charge of driving a train after a myocardial infarction.

8. FALSE   FALSE   TRUE   TRUE   FALSE

The sinoatrial node is situated at the junction of the superior vena cava and right atrium, is under the influence of sympathetic and parasympathetic fibres, is supplied in one third of cases by the circumflex coronary artery, but transmits impulses in such a way that the atria contract slightly asynchronously — the left after the right — resulting in the slightly bifid appearance of the normal P wave. There is no scientific evidence that bile salts cause bradycardia — the majority of patients with obstructive jaundice have a normal sinus rate.

9. TRUE   TRUE   FALSE   TRUE   FALSE

Repolarization changes on the ECG may follow heavy meals, biliary colic, duodenal ulceration (but not diverticular disease) and may occur in normal negroes.

Nausea, bradycardia and hypotension may follow ischaemia/infarction of the inferoposterior wall of the left ventricle in a reflex (the Bezold-Jarisch reflex) whose afferent limb is the vagus nerve, and whose efferent limb is parasympathetic vasodilator fibres and decreased sympathetic influences. This response may be abolished by atropine.

Nausea after digoxin may be a local irritant effect, or a central effect with high plasma concentrations.

PATIENT 6

Answers are on pages 32–35

HISTORY

A 24 year old secretary who is 30 weeks pregnant has been admitted from the maternity clinic with a blood pressure of 210/130 mmHg and bilateral retinal haemorrhages and exudates. Her haemoglobin is 10.9 g/dl; serum urea 10.2 mmol/l, sodium 138 mmol/l, potassium 2.6 mmol/l, and bicarbonate 31 mmol/l. There days later she goes into premature labour and is delivered of a stillborn child.

6 weeks postpartum her BP is 150/100 mmHg on no drugs, and she feels well. Her haemoglobin is now 12.8 g/dl and biochemical results from a serum sample are urea 4.2 mmol/l, sodium 138 mmol/l, potassium 3.2 mmol/l, and bicarbonate 30 mmol/l. She and her husband are keen to try again to have a child.

QUESTIONS

1. What advice would you offer?

2. What is the likely explanation of the electrolyte picture prior to delivery?

3. Would you investigate further at this juncture? If so, what investigations are indicated?

GREY CASES 31

Multiple choice questions

4. In hypertension during pregnancy:

(a) encephalopathic fits may occur with diastolic pressures less than 120 mmHg

(b) eclampsia may occur for the first time several days postpartum

(c) the use of methyldopa may lead to mental deficiency in the child

(d) fibromuscular hyperplasia of the renal arteries is a relatively common finding

(e) it may take 6 months for blood pressure to return to normal postpartum.

5. During pregnancy:

(a) plasma renin concentration rises

(b) plasma volume remains constant

(c) plasma prostaglandin E concentration rises

(d) plasma creatinine concentration rises

(e) plasma cortisol concentration rises

6. Use of the oestrogen containing oral contraceptive pill:

(a) rarely raises blood pressure before the age of 35 years

(b) is associated with an increased risk of stroke at all ages

(c) produces secondary hyperaldosteronism

(d) is contraindicated in a patient with hypercholesterolaemia

(e) may produce left ventricular hypertrophy in the absence of a rise in blood pressure.

7. In patients with primary hyperaldosteronism:

(a) the adrenal tumour is always benign

(b) plasma sodium concentration is usually high but total body sodium content is usually normal

(c) the BP and electrolyte response to spironolactone is a useful predictor of the outcome of surgery

(d) computerized tomography is a useful non invasive technique for detecting tumours less than 1 cm in diameter

(e) administration of thiazide diuretics can precipitate marked hypokalaemia and weakness

8. Reasons for failure of spironolactone to control blood pressure in some patients with primary hyperaldosteronism include:

(a) intolerable gastric side effects of the drug

(b) fluid retention

(c) associated renal impairment

(d) the hyperaldosteronism may be due to the autonomous hypersecretion of another adrenal cortical steroid

(e) simultaneous regular ingestion of aspirin

ANSWERS AND DISCUSSION

PATIENT 6

1. You should advise against further pregnancy at this juncture. BP is still elevated and further toxaemia would be likely should the patient become pregnant again. In advising about forms of contraception the oral contraceptive pill is strongly contraindicated.

2. The electrolyte picture could be indicative of secondary hyperaldosteronism related to malignant phase hypertension, but primary hyperaldosteronism cannot be excluded from these values.

3. It is still too early at 6 weeks postpartum to make an accurate assessment of this patient's renin angiotensin aldosterone system free from the effects of pregnancy. Further investigation should be delayed until at least 3, and ideally 6 months after delivery. In view of the electrolyte picture at 6 weeks postpartum primary hyperaldosteronism is a likely possibility, and further assessment of plasma renin angiotensin II and aldosterone levels, plasma and total body exchangeable sodium and potassium levels, and computerized tomography of the adrenal glands complemented, if desired, by adrenal venography and adrenal vein sampling is indicated. The blood pressure, hormone and electrolyte response to aldosterone antagonists such as spironolactone will also be of value.

4. TRUE TRUE FALSE TRUE TRUE

As with malignant phase hypertension unrelated to pregnancy hypertensive encephalopathy may occur in patients with diastolic pressures less than 120 mmHg, and is dependent on the rapidity of the rise in pressure rather than on the absolute level reached. Pre-eclampsia does not always immediately recede at delivery and eclampsia may occur for the first time in the first few days postpartum. Methyldopa has been shown to be associated with a decreased biparietal diameter in infants of mothers taking the drug through much of pregnancy, but these children do not have impaired intelligence or any other abnormality of note compared with control populations. Fibromuscular hyperplasia is the commonest cause of renal artery stenosis in young women, and appears to be commoner in parous than nulliparous patients: some workers have proposed that the relationship reflects stretching of the renal arteries during pregnancy but the mechanism is unproven. Blood pressure may take many months to return to normal in patients hypertensive during pregnancy.

5. TRUE FALSE TRUE FALSE TRUE

Physiological changes during pregnancy include a rise in both intravascular and extravascular volume along with a fall in plasma urea and creatinine concentrations and, if anything, a rise in creatinine clearance. The renin angiotensin aldosterone axis is also turned on during normal pregnancy with plasma concentrations often two or more times those occurring before and after pregnancy. Much of the rise in plasma renin is in the form of inactive renin, a larger molecule than active renin, and it is thought that much of this arises from trophoblastic tissue in the placenta. Plasma prostaglandin E concentrations are also known to rise in normal pregnancy and may play a part in governing the rise in angiotensin levels. Plasma cortisol levels rise mainly as a result of a rise in the concentration of plasma carrier protein (transcortin).

6. FALSE TRUE TRUE TRUE FALSE

The oestrogen-containing oral contraceptive pill raises blood pressure by small but significant amounts in the majority of women at all ages, even where that rise may occur within the accepted normal range. Cerebral haemorrhage and subarachnoid haemorrhage are recognized complications. Oral contraceptives should be prescribed with the greatest of caution (and should preferably be avoided) where there is present a significant risk factor or factors for vascular disease such as hypercholesterolaemia. The pill does not produce isolated left ventricular hypertrophy, but the likelist mode of action of elevation of blood pressure is through the renin angiotensin aldosterone system and secondary hyperaldosteronism is well documented.

7. FALSE FALSE TRUE FALSE TRUE

Around 1% of adrenal cortical tumours associated with primary hyperaldosteronism are malignant, and this is a lesser but nevertheless significant factor in assessing the suitability of patients for adrenalectomy. In primary hyperaldosteronism plasma and total exchangeable or total body sodium, are usually high, while the opposite is true of plasma and exchangeable potassium values. Thiazide diuretics may unmask the syndrome by precipitating profound symptomatic hypokalaemia. Computerized tomography of the adrenal areas is a useful non invasive test for identifying adrenal tumours but the current limits of resolution of the technique are around 1 cm. Thus adrenal venography and adrenal vein sampling are still far from outmoded investigations. The response of the patient to administration of aldosterone antagonists such as spironolactone is a useful predictor of the likely level of blood pressure after adrenalectomy.

8. TRUE FALSE TRUE TRUE FALSE

Spironolactone unfortunately has frequent gastric side effects such as nausea and epigastric discomfort and may even cause gastric ulceration. Spironolactone clears, not causes, fluid retention. Impairment of renal function may imply that the elevated blood pressure has been present for a long time and that irreversible changes throughout the vasculature have occurred; correction of the initial problem such as primary hyperaldosteronism will then not correct the blood pressure. There are rare but interesting cases where primary hyperaldosteronism is caused by the elaboration of an adrenocortical steroid other than aldosterone but with comparable mineralocorticoid properties; the effects of such autonomous nodules may be suppressed by dexamethasone. Ingestion of aspirin has no relevance to spironolactone therapy.

PATIENT 7

Answers are on pages 39–41

HISTORY

A 68 year old retired builder presents with a 30 minute episode of left upper arm heaviness and discomfort in his jaws following trimming of his garden hedge. He has experienced two episodes of similar character and duration over the previous 4 months, but has not sought medical help previously. On this occasion he also felt dyspnoeic and lightheaded, but did not lose consciousness. Ten years previously he underwent oversewing of a bleeding duodenal ulcer, and he also gives a 20 year history of obstructive airway disease. He has smoked 30 cigarettes daily for over 50 years, and currently takes slow-release salbutamol 8 mg at night, and salbutamol inhaler 2 puffs four times daily.

EXAMINATION

On examination he is small and thin with a fine tremor of outstretched hands. Respiratory — poor chest expansion; resonant percussion note; no crepitations; bilateral rhonchi. Cardiovascular — blood pressure 130/80 mmHg in the right arm lying; pulse 95/min, regular; apex beat in the sixth intercostal space 2 cm outwith the midclavicular line; fourth heart sound present; no murmurs. Neurological examination normal.

Chest X-ray — emphysema: cardiothoracic ratio — 160:280.
ECG — sinus rhythm: left ventricular hypertrophy and strain (SVI + RV6 = 54 mm).

QUESTIONS

1. What explanations for his presentation would you consider?

2. What explanations can you offer for the ECG findings?

3. Which three blood tests would you find most helpful?

4. Which two non invasive tests will help you most to arrive at a diagnosis?

Multiple choice questions

5. With regard to the management of hypothyroidism which of the following statements is/are correct?
(a) *Resting pulse rate is a reliable index of the adequacy of thyroxine replacement therapy*
(b) *Coarse hair, dry skin, hoarse voice, and sinus rhythm 76/minute are not compatible with untreated thyrotoxicosis*
(c) *Premenopausal hypothyroid women are relatively protected against the contribution of myxoedema to coronary artery disease*
(d) *Obesity occurring as part of the consequences of hypothyroidism is an important independent risk factor for coronary artery disease*
(e) *Thyroxine 0.1 mg once daily is a dangerous starting dose for thyroid replacement therapy*

6. In **adults** with aortic stenosis:
(a) *angina pectoris may be due to calcification of the proximal left main coronary artery*

(b) *valvotomy is indicated when dyspnoea becomes severe*

(c) *a characteristic finding is a small volume jerky pulse*

(d) *left ventricular hypertrophy usually resolves in the 6 months after aortic valve replacement*

(e) *aggressive behaviour may be an important sign of preterminal aortic valve disease*

7. Which of the following statements is/are true?

(a) *A peak systolic gradient of 10 mmHg across the aortic valve indicates significant aortic stenosis*

(b) *The absence of a systolic gradient across the aortic valve satisfactorily excludes a diagnosis of hypertrophic cardiomyopathy*

(c) *A systolic gradient of 20 mmHg across an aortic valve prosthesis does not call for any action*

(d) *A jugular venous pulse 5 cm above the angle of Louis is synonymous with right atrial pressure of 5 mmHg*

(e) *At cardiac catheterization the left atrium is often catheterized retrogradely via the mitral valve*

8. Which of the following statements is/are true?

(a) *The main venous drainage of the heart is by the coronary sinus to the right ventricle*

(b) *The left circumflex coronary artery runs in the left atrioventricular groove to supply the atrioventricular node in the majority of cases*

(c) *The left main coronary artery may be short, but is always present in the left atrioventricular groove*

(d) *The left anterior and posterior hemibundles are clearly distinguishable in the majority of autopsy specimens*

(e) *The largest valvar ring belongs to the mitral valve*

9. Symptoms of congestive cardiac failure include:

(a) *anorexia*

(b) *insomnia*

(c) *exophthalmos*

(d) *weakness of limbs*

(e) *menorrhagia.*

ANSWERS AND DISCUSSION

PATIENT 7

1. The patient's presenting symptoms are characteristic of myocardial ischaemia/infarction secondary to (a) coronary artery disease; or (b) transient bradyarrhythmia; or (c) transient tachyarrhythmia — possible contributory factors include sympathomimetic overdosage, occult thyrotoxicosis, silent aortic stenosis, and anaemia following further gastrointestinal blood loss, acute or chronic.

2. (a) Prior hypertension — current relative hypotension after myocardial infarction, or gastrointestinal bleed.
(b) Aortic stenosis with a clinically undetectable murmur, indicating severe outflow obstruction.
(c) Hypertrophic cardiomyopathy — less likely in view of the patient's age and absence of other symptoms.
(d) Ischaemic cardiomyopathy — poorly functioning dilated left ventricle, with or without hypertrophy of remaining healthy myocardium.

3. Cardiac enzymes, serum thyroxine (or result of TRH test), and haemoglobin (looking for polycythaemia, or anaemia) would be most helpful.

4. A 24 hour ECG recording, and an echocardiogram would be most helpful.

5. FALSE   FALSE   FALSE   FALSE   TRUE

Pulse rate is an unreliable index in patients who may also have ischaemic heart disease and may be receiving beta-blockers — a TSH level is the most valuable index. In 'apathetic' thyrotoxicosis the symptoms and physical appearance particularly in elderly patients may suggest hypothyroidism, but blood tests reveal the true diagnosis. Premenopausal women are not protected from the atherogenic effects of myxoedema; obesity is a relatively unimportant risk factor in its own right. Myocardial ischaemia/infarction may be precipitated even at starting doses of 50 μg thyroxine on alternate days — 0.1 mg thyroxine daily is dangerous initially.

6. TRUE   FALSE   FALSE   FALSE   TRUE

Calcific aortic stenosis may involve the proximal coronary arteries in calcification: valvotomy is a hazardous procedure liable to produce torrential regurgitation and rapid demise. A jerky small volume pulse is characteristic of hypertrophic cardiomyopathy where initial vigorous expulsion of blood from the left ventricle is arrested by outflow tract obstruction. Left ventricular hypertrophy may take years to resolve though early ECG changes may be striking — an aortic prosthesis, however, usually constitutes continuing mild obstruction. Angina pectoris, exertional syncope and arrhythmic symptoms are characteristic of aortic stenosis, but where cardiac output is persistently very low symptoms of cerebral hypoxia at rest may be prominent.

7. FALSE   FALSE   TRUE   FALSE   FALSE

A 10 mmHg systolic gradient across the aortic valve is trivial, and a 20 mmHg gradient across an aortic prosthesis expected. In hypertrophic cardiomyopathy the outflow obstruction may be low in the outflow tract, there being no gradient across the valve itself. Retrograde catheterization of the left atrium via the mitral valve would be a happy accident. To the vertical height of the JVP above the angle of Louis, a further 5 cm on average must be added to give the true central venous pressure.

8. FALSE FALSE FALSE FALSE FALSE

The coronary sinus drains into the right atrium. In 90% of cases the AV node is supplied by a terminal branch of the right coronary artery. The left anterior descending and circumflex arteries may have separate origins in the left sinus of Valsalva. Hemibundles are a convenient ECG convention but comparable anatomical structures are not commonly identified. The tricuspid, mitral, pulmonary and aortic valves have supporting rings with dimensions of decreasing magnitude.

9. TRUE TRUE FALSE TRUE FALSE

Symptoms of congestive cardiac failure include fatigue and weakness, cerebral symptoms such as nightmares and insomnia, and anorexia (gut oedema may be contributory). It should be noted however that these may all be side-effects of possibly related drugs, respectively hyponatraemia with diuretics, cerebral symptoms with beta-blockers, and anorexia with digoxin.

PATIENT 8

Answers are on pages 44–46

HISTORY

A 47 year old miner has been admitted to the coronary care unit 36 hours previously with a characteristic history of prolonged retrosternal discomfort radiating to both shoulders. ECGs have demonstrated changes of an evolving anteroseptal myocardial infarction, while the CPK-MB 24 hours after admission is 1350 U/1. You have been called to see him because the staff nurse has recorded his temperature as 38.8°C, though the patient is uncomplaining.

QUESTIONS

1. What is your differential diagnosis?

2. The white cell count is 11.5×10^9/l while the ESR is 60 mm in the first hour. Which of your differential diagnoses do/does these findings support?

You are unable to detect any abnormalities on physical examination. 4 hours later you are called to visit the patient urgently. He is now moribund — hypotensive and cyanosed — and dies within 5 minutes though not of an arrhythmia.

3. What cause(s) of death do you suspect?

Multiple choice questions

4. In the Frank-Starling curve of stroke volume against left ventricular filling pressure;

(a) *intravenous nitrates shift the curve down and to the right*

(b) *giving nitrate will always reduce filling pressure while maintaining stroke volume constant*

(c) *increased myocardial contractility shifts the curve upwards and to the left*

(d) *the greater the filling pressure the higher the stroke volume*

(e) *administration of nifedipine may shift the curve upwards.*

5. Pulmonary oedema:

(a) *may be relieved by morphine reducing preload on the heart*

(b) *may be the presenting feature of subarachnoid haemorrhage*

(c) *always implies left ventricular failure*

(d) *is common in patients with atrial septal defect*

(e) *may follow inhalation of chlorine gas*

6. Sinus bradycardia may be caused by:

(a) *anaesthesia*

(b) *raised intracranial pressure*

(c) *acute intravascular volume depletion*

(d) *digoxin*

(e) *pericardial effusion.*

7. Following a myocardial infarction:

(a) *digoxin should be discontinued before discharge from hospital if atrial fibrillation occurred briefly in the coronary care unit*

(b) *a positive exercise test performed 6 weeks post-infarct indicates disease in a coronary artery other than that supplying the infarcted area*

(c) patients should be anticoagulated for 3 months

(d) there are no restrictions which should be imposed on driving a private car

(e) fasting lipid estimations should be delayed for several weeks.

8. The following may cause myocardial infarction, independent of atheroma:

(a) infective endocarditis of the mitral valve

(b) road traffic accident

(c) mural thrombus of the left ventricle

(d) polyarteritis nodosa

(e) carbon monoxide poisoning.

ANSWERS AND DISCUSSION

PATIENT 8

1. Tissue (myocardial) necrosis.
Pericarditis.
Respiratory infection.
Urinary tract infection (especially if catheterised).
Deep venous thrombosis.

2. A rapid ESR and leucocytosis exclude none of the differential diagnoses.

3. Extension of myocardial infarction or second myocardial infarction with pump failure.
Myocardial rupture.
Stroke from mural thrombus.

Pulmonary embolism, though sinus tachycardia or atrial fibrillation would be expected.

4. FALSE   TRUE   TRUE   FALSE   TRUE

Nitrates are predominantly venodilators and reduce preload, thereby shifting the curve to the left, but leaving cardiac output unaltered. Improved myocardial contractility shifts the curve upwards and to the left. Administration of nifedipine, an arteriolar vasodilator, reduces afterload and shifts the curve upwards. Within limits the greater the filling pressure the greater the stroke volume, but if the left ventricle is overdilated, cardiac output falls off again.

5. TRUE   TRUE   FALSE   FALSE   TRUE

As well as central sedative effects morphine has important venodilator and arteriolar effects. Pulmonary oedema may be caused by imbalance of Starling forces as in left ventricular failure, altered alveolar-capillary membrane permeability as in chlorine inhalation, lymphatic disease such as lymphangitis carcinomatosis, and a variety of ill understood causes such as sudden elevation to high altitude, a variety of neurological problems including subrarachnoid haemorrhage, and after cardiopulmonary bypass. Unless there is associated ischaemic heart disease, hypertension or valvular disease left ventricular failure would be unlikely in patients with atrial septal defect, and even if this does occur increased shunting and a presentation with right heart failure is more likely.

6. TRUE   TRUE   FALSE   TRUE   FALSE

By a variety of vagal influences anaesthesia may produce bradycardia. Sudden elevations in intracranial pressure may produce the Cushing response with bradycardia and hypertension. Digoxin toxicity numbers sinus bradycardia among its many effects. Acute hypovolaemia causes tachycardia, as does pericardial effusion.

7. TRUE   TRUE   FALSE   FALSE   TRUE

Transient atrial fibrillation during an acute ischaemic episode is no reason for long term digoxin administration. A positive exercise test is a helpful indicator of coronary artery disease more widespread than the vessel supplying the infarcted area. The place of routine anticoagulation remains to be established, and where it is employed as a routine there is no evidence that it should be continued once the patient is mobile. Fasting lipid estimation to be truly accurate should be delayed for several weeks, since marked elevations may occur during any illness. Advice regarding avoidance of driving for two months after the infarction, and completely if angina is easily provoked by driving, is sound.

8. TRUE   TRUE   TRUE   TRUE   TRUE

It is important to remember that myocardial infarction has causes other than atherosclerosis — emboli (infective, thrombotic, neoplastic or fat); arteritis (such as polyarteritis nodosa); metabolic disorders (such as homocystinuria); trauma; narrowing of the orifice of a coronary artery as in dissection of the aorta; coronary artery spasm; congenital anomalies of the coronary arteries; aortic valve disease; thyrotoxicosis; carbon monoxide poisoning; and the well documented syndrome of myocardial infarction with normal coronary arteries and no demonstrable cause.

PATIENT 9

Answers are on pages 50–52

HISTORY

A 50 year old woman is referred by her general practitioner for advice regarding the management of her hypertension: this has been treated with bendrofluazide 10 mg o.d. and clonidine 0.3 mg t.i.d. for 5 years with BP recordings varying from 120/70 to 210/134 mmHg. Over the previous 6 months the patient has developed episodes of chest tightness on exertion, lasting 10 minutes, and relieved by rest and glyceryl trinitrate. She has, in addition, a 25 year history of bronchial asthma with sensitivity to house dust mite, feathers and cat fur: for this she is currently receiving prednisolone 7.5 mg daily orally and salbutamol inhaler two puffs q.i.d. Despite many injunctions to the contrary she has continued to smoke 20 cigarettes daily, and over a 2 year period she has had three severe episodes of bronchospasm precipitated by chest infection; during the last two attacks she has failed to use prophylactic antibiotics left for her by her general practitioner.

EXAMINATION

On examination the patient is thin, plethoric, and has a hyperresonant chest with an audible wheeze. BP 194/128 mmHg lying, 180/122 mmHg standing with optic fundal examination showing arteriovenous nipping but no haemorrhages or exudates. Pulse 86/min regular. Heart sounds normal. 24 hours later her BP has fallen to 130/96 mmHg. Full blood count and serum urea and electrolytes are normal.

QUESTIONS

1. From the available information what possible causes of this patient's hypertension are likely?

2. What explanation can you offer for the variable BP recordings?

3. What would be your (a) initial and (b) longterm drug therapy, and what are your reasons for your choices?

4. Do you think further investigation is indicated?

Multiple choice questions

5. The following conditions constitute relative contraindications to the use of the named drugs:

(a) *maturity onset diabetes mellitus (R_x glibenclamide and diet) — metoprolol*

(b) *cirrhosis of the liver — methyldopa*

(c) *epilepsy — prazosin*

(d) *scleroderma — hydrallazine*

(e) *gout — debrisoquine.*

6. In hypertensive patients with Cushing's syndrome it is not unusual to find:

(a) *truncal obesity*

(b) *hyponatraemia*

(c) *psychiatric illness*

(d) *loss of height*

(e) *pericardial effusion.*

7. Prolonged blood pressure elevation may be caused by the longterm administration of:

(a) *methyltestosterone*

(b) *methylprenisolone*

(c) *dexamethasone*

(d) *indomethacin*

(e) *carbenoxolone.*

8. Beta-adrenergic neurone blocking drugs have been used extensively in the treatment of hypertension.

(a) *They are the drug of first choice in patients with Conn's syndrome.*

(b) *They may impair renal function.*

(c) *They often precipitate cardiac failure in the presence of renal dysfunction.*

(d) *They are the drug of first choice in hypertensive patients with angina pectoris.*

(e) *Cardioselective beta-blockers do not cause significant airways obstruction.*

5. When a hypertensive patient previously well controlled on a combination of atenolol bendrofluazide and prazosin is found to have an unexpected rise in blood pressure the following may be relevant investigations:

(a) *pulse rate response to exercise*

(b) *plasma albumin*

(c) *plasma glucose concentration*

(d) *renal arteriography*

(e) *urinary normetadrenaline concentration.*

ANSWERS AND DISCUSSION

PATIENT 9

1. Essential hypertension
Steroid induced hypertension
Phaeochromocytoma

2. Phaeochromocytoma attacks but symptomatology is lacking. Erratic clonidine ingestion producing phaemochromocytoma like attacks. Non-compliance with prescribed therapy unrelated to the clonidine withdrawal syndrome.

3. (a) Initial — labetalol or phenoxybenzamine/beta-blocker combination are relatively contraindicated because of the severe respiratory disease. Clonidine, however, must be withdrawn in this patient because erratic compliance could be lethal. Ideally gradual weaning of the patient from clonidine under inpatient supervision is required.
(b) Longterm — diuretics alone may be sufficient to control this patient's blood pressure. Nifedipine would then be the ideal drug to introduce because of its antihypertensive and anti-anginal effects, and also because of the relative protection it affords against bronchoconstriction.

4. Yes — identification of a correctable cause for this patient's hypertension is the ideal alternative to drug treatment in a non compliant patient. However, the hypertension is of long standing and removal of the primary cause,, should one be identified at this late stage, may not return blood pressure to normal; it may, however, make it easier to control.

5. TRUE   TRUE   FALSE   TRUE   FALSE

Metoprolol will partially mask the signs and symptoms of

hypoglycaemia which may be precipitated by an inappropriate combination of diet and glibenclamide. Methyldopa may cause liver enzyme abnormalities and occasionally overt hepatitis in its own right and is best avoided in a patient with underlying hepatic dysfunction. Prazosin rarely causes hypotensive collapse but this does not constitute a significant contraindication to its use in an epileptic patient. Since hydrallazine quite commonly produces disturbances of antinuclear factor though less commonly causes overt systemic lupus erythematosus its use in a patient with an allied collagen disorder is contraindicated; furthermore the hypertension associated with scleroderma is usually of an intractable nature and often responds only to minoxidil or captopril. Debrisoquine is not associated with hyperuricaemia.

6. TRUE FALSE TRUE TRUE FALSE

Recognized features of Cushing's syndrome include truncal obesity with slender extremities and proximal muscle weakness, hypertension (in 80-90%), diabetes mellitus (in approximately 20%), hirsutism, amenorrhoea, deepening of the voice, emotional lability or even frank psychosis, and osteoporosis affecting mainly the spine and pelvis and sometimes associated with vertebral body collapse and loss of height, hypokalaemia with usually normal plasma sodium concentrations but occasionally hypernatraemia. Pericardial effusion is not a direct effect of the glucocorticoid, androgen or mineralocorticoid excess.

7. FALSE TRUE TRUE TRUE TRUE

Iatrogenic hypertension may be caused by administration of methylprednisolone and dexamethasone (glucocorticoid effect), carbenoxolone (mineralocorticoid effect) and by indomethacin (salt and water retention).

8. FALSE TRUE FALSE TRUE FALSE

Spironolactone is the drug of first choice in primary hyperaldosteronism though beta blockers may be helpful in addition if spironolactone alone is unsuccessful. A 10-15% reduction in renal blood flow has been shown to follow administration of propranolol by some workers. The presence of renal dysfunction does not imply that betablockers will precipitate cardiac failure. In the absence of any contraindication such as severe chronic obstructive airways disease beta-blockers are the drug of first choice in a patient with both hypertension and angina pectoris; a further useful drug is nifedipine. Cardioselective beta-blockers are not completely selective though they undoubtedly have less in the way of respiratory side effects; they are nevertheless best avoided if possible in patients with a history of airways obstruction.

9. TRUE   FALSE   FALSE   TRUE   FALSE

A brisk increase in pulse rate with exercise suggests that the patient is receiving inadequate beta-blockers and in view of the previous good control this suggests poor current compliance with therapy. Plasma albumin and glucose concentrations are peripheral investigations and do not provide a ready explanation of the deterioration in control, nor are urinary normetadrenaline concentrations a discriminating test in these circumstances. Renal arteriography, however, in a compliant patent may show the development of a renal artery stenosis as the cause of the BP rise.

PATIENT 10

Answers are on pages 55–57

HISTORY

A 65 year old man presents to the cardiology outpatient clinic complaining of nausea, flatulence and anorexia of 4 weeks' standing. He suffered three attacks of rheumatic fever in his 'teens with subsequent rheumatic valvular heart disease. 8 years previously his mitral valve was replaced with a Starr-Edwards prosthesis while 8 weeks previously, following a deterioration in anginal symptoms and in congestive cardiac failure, he underwent an uncomplicated aortic valve replacement with a further Starr-Edwards prosthesis. His regular medication consists of digoxin 0.25 mg o.d., frusemide 40 mg o.d., warfarin and potassium supplements.

EXAMINATION

On examination he is mildly icteric. BP 144/92 mmHg in right arm, lying. Pulse — atrial fibrillation with a ventricular rate of 50/minute, normal volume. Native and prosthetic sounds normal. Soft systolic murmurs at base and apex but no diastolic murmurs. JVP + 8 cm above angle of Louis. Slight pitting ankle oedema bilaterally. Bilateral basal crepitations. 6 cm smooth hepatomegaly.
Urinalysis: Protein +. Bilirubin ++. Urobilinogen ++.

QUESTIONS

1. How can you explain this patient's complaints of (a) nausea, (b) hepatomegaly and (c) jaundice?

2. Which four blood tests will you find most helpful in establishing the diagnosis?

Multiple choice questions

3. Longterm warfarin therapy is indicated in the longterm management of adult patients with:

(a) *porcine heterograft valves*

(b) *atrial septal defect*

(c) *paroxysmal ventricular tachycardia*

(d) *mitral stenosis but sinus rhythm*

(e) *atrial fibrillation secondary to thyrotoxicosis.*

4. The dosage of warfarin must be adjusted following the introduction of:

(a) *prednisolone*

(b) *dihydrocodeine*

(c) *cholestyramine*

(d) *amiodarone*

(e) *oral contraceptives.*

5. Following aortic valve replacement:

(a) *angina pectoris may resolve*

(b) *complete heart block is a common late finding*

(c) *a soft early diastolic murmur may safely be ignored*

(d) *the occurrence of acute pulmonary oedema is most likely to indicate acute myocardial infarction*

(e) *persistent pyrexia warrants investigation for SLE.*

6. Complications of temporary right ventricular pacing include:

(a) *haemopericardium*

(b) *hiccoughs*

(c) *pulmonary oedema*

(d) *atrial fibrillation*

(e) *surgical emphysema.*

7. Which of the following statements is/are true?

(a) *Warfarin is largely protein bound.*

(b) *Where anticoagulant control with warfarin is poor nicoumalone may be of benefit.*

(c) *Warfarin may produce liver dysfunction.*

(d) *Anticoagulation is desirable before venography of the calf veins.*

(e) *Skin rash is one of the commoner side-effects of warfarin.*

ANSWERS AND DISCUSSION

PATIENT 10

1. (a) Nausea may have been caused by digoxin toxicity, jaundice, right heart failure with hepatic congestion, or viral hepatitis. In the context of recent cardiac surgery and multiple transfusions you should be particularly concerned about hepatitis B or cytomegalovirus hepatitis.
   (b) Hepatomegaly could be the result of viral hepatitis or congestive cardiac failure.

(c) Jaundice may be due to hepatitis or hepatic congestion (right heart failure) but haemolysis in a patient with two Starr-Edwards prostheses is an important contributorry factor (note urobilinogen in urine).

2. Reticulocyte count (haemolysis)
Viral antibodies
Liver function tests
Digoxin assay

3. FALSE   FALSE   FALSE   TRUE   TRUE

Systemic embolism is not a common accompaniment of atrial septal defect, and it occurs only occasionally in paroxysmal V.T. With heterograft valves, providing the patient is in sinus rhythm, the hazards of warfarin therapy outweight advantages of anticoagulation after the first 3 months. Not all patients with mitral stenosis require warfarin, particularly where a patient in sinus rhythm has undergone mitral valvotomy and may be looking forward to decades of good health, but where the stenosis is tightening anticoagulants are indicated even where the patient remains in sinus rhythm. Until a patient is euthyroid anticoagulation in hyperthyroidism may be necessary where embolism has occurred, but as a routine it is not prescribed to toxic patients in sinus rhythm.

4. TRUE   TRUE   TRUE   TRUE   TRUE

Many drugs interfere with warfarin absorption (cholestyramine), metabolism (barbiturate) or protein binding (amiodarone). The dangers of combining warfarin and amiodarone have recently been recognized as have combining digoxin and amiodarone and it is important since the combination is becoming common in the management of paroxysmal supraventricular tachycardia.

5. TRUE   TRUE   FALSE   FALSE   FALSE

With regression of left ventricular hypertrophy and improved output through the coronary arteries after aortic valve replacement, angina may resolve. Damage to the conducting system is a common early complication, and calcification of the conducting pathways not a rare later problem. Paraprosthetic leaks (diastolic murmurs) are potentially very hazardous, as is mechanical blockade of the prosthesis, by thrombus for example, resulting in acute pulmonary oedema. The initials used are SLE not SBE.

6. TRUE   TRUE   TRUE   TRUE   TRUE

Complications may accompany any part of the procedure of temporary pacemaker insertion. Subclavian vein puncture may inadvertently cause apical lung puncture with surgical emphysema. Passage of the electrode may induce (usually transient) atrial ectopics or fibrillation, and ventricular ectopics tachycardia or fibrillation. Penetration of soft myocardium by the electrode may produce pericarditis and rarely mild haemopericardium; rarely this may stimulate the phrenic nerve with rapid regular hiccoughing, as may displacement of the electrode to the inferior vena cava at the level of the diaphragm. Temporary pacing may also induce pulmonary oedema, if the contribution of the atrial 'kick' to cardiac output is lost in a patient with borderline cardiac failure.

7. TRUE   TRUE   TRUE   TRUE   TRUE

The protein binding of warfarin is one of the main factors contributing to potentiation of the drug's activity when combined with other protein bound agents. For ill understood reasons substitution of nicoumalone which has little pharmacological difference to warfarin may be helpful in gaining good anticoagulant control. In its own right warfarin may induce a maculopapular skin eruption and also, rarely, liver dysfunction. Heparin on the other hand is a desirable anticoagulant if a patient with suspected deep venous thrombosis is going to undergo venography (a thrombogenic procedure) the following day.

PATIENT 11

Answers are on pages 61–63

HISTORY

A 24 year old girl was known to have a normal blood pressure (126/80 mmHg) when she was started on the oestrogen-containing oral contraceptive pill at a family planning clinic.

3 months later, while on holiday, she developed severe headache with visual disturbance and was admitted to hospital after several grand mal seizures. Her BP was 260/160 mmHg and she had bilateral optic fundal haemorrhages exudates and papilloedema. Her BP was controlled with intravenous nitroprusside and she was referred for further investigation. Her past medical history consisted only of occasional urinary tract infections in childhood. Examination apart from the above findings was normal.

INITIAL INVESTIGATION

Haemoglobin 10.4 g/dl, reticulocytes 2.6%, white cell count 10.1×10^9/l, serum sodium concn 133 mmol/l, potassium 3.6 mmol/l, bicarbonate 29 mmol/l, urea 12.1 mmol/l. At intravenous urography there was absence of contrast in the right kidney at 3 minutes after the injection of contrast: at 20 minutes contrast was absent from the left kidney but present on the right.

QUESTIONS

1. What is the likely diagnosis?

2. (a) What is the explanation of the blood findings?
   (b) What three other blood tests could usefully be performed to clarify the position?

3. What further noninvasive test would be helpful in clarifying the renal abnormality?

4. Renal arteriography surprisingly was normal, but the renal vein renin ratio was 1.7:1. In view of these findings what is the likely aetiology of the hypertension?

Multiple choice questions

5. In malignant phase hypertension:

(a) *there is, untreated, a 50% mortality at 2 years*

(b) *rapid blood pressure control by parenteral drug therapy is desirable*

(c) *once blood pressure has been controlled papilloedema resolves quickly*

(d) *abdominal pain may be the presenting symptom*

(e) *nocturia is a common complaint.*

6. The finding of a normal plasma angiotensin II concentration in a patient with hypertension suspected to be due to renal artery stenosis:

(a) *precludes a cause and effect relationship between the stenosis and the hypertension*

(b) *implies that the patient is in acute renal failure*

(c) *implies that the patient is taking diuretics*

(d) *is common*

(e) *is likely if the patient is being treated with oral converting enzyme inhibitors.*

7. Intravenous urography:

(a) yields a high percentage of abnormal results in screening of the hypertensive population
(b) can precipitate acute renal failure in diabetics
(c) may cause fatal anaphylaxis
(d) in patients with renal artery stenosis, produces a picture where contrast is absent from the affected kidney in later films
(e) should be performed with frequent films in the first 5 minutes after injection of contrast to aid in the detection of renal artery stenosis.

8. The finding of renal artery stenosis in a hypertensive patient:

(a) may be coincidental
(b) may be the result rather than the cause of the hypertension
(c) together with a renal vein renin ratio greater than 2.0 implies that a successful outcome from renovascular surgery is likely
(d) infers that coronary and cerebral artery disease is likely to be present
(e) is a less common potentially correctable finding than an adrenal adenoma.

9. Recognized complications of parenteral administration of the following hypotensive agents are:

(a) tingling of the scalp — labetalol
(b) myocardial infarction — diazoxide
(c) hypothyroidism — nitroprusside
(d) a rise in blood pressure — clonidine
(e) nausea and vomiting — hydrallazine.

ANSWERS AND DISCUSSION

PATIENT 11

1. Malignant phase hypertension secondary to right renal artery stenosis.

2. (a) Microangiopathic haemolytic anaemia secondary to the malignant phase hypertension.
(b) Blood film looking for evidence of red cell fragmentation, platelet count and fibrin degradation products.

3. ^{123}I or ^{131}I hippuran renography.

4. It is likely that ischaemic damage to small vessels (fibrinoid necrosis) resulting from the malignant phase hypertension has produced the picture of right renal ischaemia. In view of the temporal relationship between starting the oral contraceptive pill and the discovery of the malignant phase hypertension it is likely that this girl's illness has been precipitated by the oral contraceptive pill. With control of her blood pressure much of this ischaemic damage may resolve.

5. FALSE   FALSE   FALSE   TRUE   TRUE

The mortality rate is of the order of 90% at 2 years in patients with untreated malignant phase hypertension. Blood pressure need not be controlled by parenteral means unless complications such as hypertensive left heart failure or encephalopathy is present, since rapid BP reduction may precipitate potentially lethal myocardial ischaemia/infarction or cerebral infarction; of the available parenteral therapies labetalol appears to be associated with the least sinister side effects. Once BP has been controlled the optic fundal abnormalities may take weeks or months to resolve. Symptoms, when present, are usually of headache or visual disturbance, though nocturia is not uncommon; abdominal pain is a less common but recognised symptom indicating either the underlying cause of the hypertension such as renal infarction, or the consequence of fibrinoid necrosis producing bowel wall infarction. Many causes of malignant phase hypertension have been identified and include ingestion of the oral contraceptive pill.

6. FALSE   FALSE   FALSE   TRUE   FALSE

Although plasma angiotensin II concentration may be raised in patients with renovascular hypertension it is commonly within the normal range; though such a finding may be consistent with a stenosis of long standing it is not necessarily so and does not preclude a successful outcome from renovascular surgery. Oral converting enzyme inhibitors produce low and often unrecordable plasma angiotensin II levels, while diuretics increase the levels, as would renal artery stenosis (usually bilateral) sufficiently severe to produce acute renal failure.

7. FALSE   TRUE   TRUE   FALSE   TRUE

Intravenous urography will give a high yield of positive results in a specialist hypertension referral unit but not in the general hypertensive population. It is not free from side effects which include anaphylaxis, local tissue reactions, and acute renal failure, partly related to fluid restriction before the test and commoner in diabetic patients with an underlying degree of renal impairment. It is useful in screening for renal artery stenosis. Frequent early (or 'minute sequence') films may demonstrate delay in the appearance of contrast on the affected side and later films may show increased density on the affected side with delay in the washout of contrast after an oral water load. Other helpful signs include a decrease in the bipolar diameter of the affected kidney, calyceal spasticity and ureteric notching. The above appearances are typical of stenosis of moderate severity; where the stenosis is severe or complete contrast may fail to appear on the affected side.

8. TRUE   TRUE   TRUE   FALSE   FALSE

When renal artery stenosis is found in a hypertensive patient (a) the stenosis may have caused the hypertension and correction of the stenosis surgically may or may not cure the hypertension (b) the hypertension may have preceded the stenosis and by contributing to the formation of atheroma may have helped form the stenosis (c) a stenosis so formed may become more severe and further increase blood pressure — successful surgery will then only return blood pressure to its previously elevated level (d) the hypertension and the stenosis are unrelated findings since both independently are common. If the renal vein renin ratio is 2.0 or greater a successful outcome from surgery is likely but not guaranteed, while a successful outcome will also occur in many patients with a ratio of less than 2.0 though it is difficult to predict which patients will respond. Stenoses of other major arteries may occur in patients with renal artery stenosis caused by both atheroma and fibromuscular hyperplasia, but the renal lesion often occurs as an isolated abnormality. Renal artery stenosis is the commonest potentially correctable cause of hypertension occurring in at least 5% of the hypertensive population compared with a figure of around 2% for adrenal adenoma.

9. TRUE   TRUE   TRUE   TRUE   TRUE

All of the effects mentioned may occur with the named drugs. Parenteral hypotensive drugs are best avoided if at all possible. The reason for the scalp tingling with labetalol is not well understood. Diazoxide produces a particularly precipitate and uncontrolled fall in pressure and has been associated with myocardial infarction. Nitroprusside, if continued for several days, interferes significantly with iodine metabolism in the thyroid gland. Parenteral clonidine may cause a paradoxical rise in blood pressure through peripheral alpha receptor stimulation. Hydrallazine in common with many of the parenteral hypotensive drugs may precipitate nausea and vomiting as blood pressure is rapidly lowered.

PATIENT 12

Answers are on pages 66–68

HISTORY

A 56 year old man is admitted to the coronary care unit for the sixth time in 12 months with burning retrosternal discomfort of 2 hours' duration, radiating to the left shoulder and arm, with its onset at rest. The discomfort is unrelieved by glyceryl trinitrate, but is relieved apparently by nifedipine 10 mg sublingually on admission to the unit. On this occasion, as on three of the previous admissions, symmetrical T wave inversion on leads V4 — V6 of the ECG is observed, but the changes resolve within 24 hours. Cardiac enzymes remain normal.

QUESTIONS

1. What is the differential diagnosis?

2. What invasive investigations, if any, would you advocate, and in what order would you perform them?

3. In the short term which medications do you consider are worthy of a clinical trial?

Multiple choice questions

4. An exercise tolerance test is contraindicated:

(a) *if the resting diastolic blood pressure is in excess of 120 mmHg*

(b) *if digoxin is being taken regularly by the patient*
(c) *in the first 3 weeks after a myocardial infarction*
(d) *in severe aortic stenosis*
(e) *in unstable angina pectoris.*

5. An exercise tolerance test should be stopped:
(a) *if the patient so wishes*
(b) *if ventricular bigeminy occurs*
(c) *if dyspnoea occurs*
(d) *if left bundle branch block occurs*
(e) *if systolic blood pressure drops during exercise.*

6. Ebstein's anomaly:
(a) *affects the mitral and tricuspid valves*
(b) *includes underdevelopment of the right ventricle*
(c) *is often associated with a ventricular septal defect*
(d) *is incompatible with normal life expectancy*
(e) *is not amenable to surgery.*

7. Indications for insertion of a temporary pacemaker after myocardial infarction include:
(a) *Mobitz Type II block*
(b) *atrial fibrillation*
(c) *right bundle branch block and left posterior hemiblock in anterior myocardial infarction*
(d) *nodal bradycardia of 50 beats/minute*
(e) *left anterior hemiblock and first degree atrioventricular block.*

8. Digoxin:
(a) *is principally absorbed from the stomach*
(b) *is contraindicated in hypertrophic cardiomyopathy*

(c) *plasma levels become stable in chronic renal failure after regular administration of the drug for 3 days*
(d) *toxicity may be reversed with digitalis antibodies*
(e) *half-life is prolonged in hypothyroidism.*

ANSWERS AND DISCUSSION

PATIENT 12

1. Coronary artery spasm.
Paroxysmal arrhythmia producing myocardial ischaemia.
Oesophageal spasm.

2. In view of the unstable nature of the patient's condition and the ECG changes coronary angiography is indicated after controlled exercise testing and 24 hour ambulatory ECG recordings. If this proves normal then oesophageal manometry after barium swallow may be helpful.

3. Sublingual glyceryl trinitrate and nifedipine may be helpful for spasm of both coronary arteries and oesophagus. If symptoms are more suggestive of gastrointestinal pathology then a trial of antacid and an antispasmodic are indicated.

4. TRUE   FALSE   FALSE   TRUE   TRUE

An exercise test is contraindicated (i) in a patient with unstable angina since no extra diagnostic information will be gained and the procedure is potentially lethal; (ii) in severe aortic stenosis where fatal syncope may ensue; (iii) and in an already hypertensive patient since blood pressure is expected to rise further during exercise. Digoxin makes interpretation of the test difficult, but diagnostic information may still be obtained. As part of the rehabilitation process, and also to look for disease in other coronary arteries, exercise testing after myocardial infarction may be very helpful.

5. TRUE   TRUE   FALSE   TRUE   TRUE

A positive test may be indicated by features other than ST segment depression — characteristic chest pain, development of bundle branch block, arrhythmia including ventricular bigeminy, and hypotension are all valid reasons to stop the test, as is the patient's disinclination to continue. The occurrence of dyspnoea alone, however, should not deter the clinician from urging the patient towards a target heart rate, unless the dyspnoea becomes distressing.

6. FALSE   TRUE   FALSE   FALSE   FALSE

Ebstein's anomaly consists of downward displacement of a malformed tricuspid valve into a variably underdeveloped right ventricle. The commonest concurrent anomalies are atrial septal defect or patent foramen ovale. The Wolff-Parkinson-White (Type B) syndrome is not uncommon, and tachyarrhythmia, atrial or ventricular, is a common problem later in the course of the disease. Many patients survive to adult life and may have a normal life expectancy. Where the condition is more severe, however, cyanosis is common and right heart failure may be the mode of death. In patients with less marked underdevelopment of the right ventricle tricuspid valve replacement with or without closure of an atrial septal defect may greatly benefit the patient.

7. TRUE   TRUE   TRUE   FALSE   FALSE

Practice is not uniform with regard to temporary pacing in acute myocardial infarction. There is evidence however that pacing is of benefit in patients with symptomatic bradycardia unresponsive to atropine, bifascicular block (RBBB + LAD or RBBB + RAD) or trifascicular block (bifascicular block or LBBB with first degree A-V block), anterior infarction with second or third degree A-V block, and documented asystolic episodes.

8. TRUE   TRUE   FALSE   TRUE   TRUE

Digoxin is rapidly absorbed from the stomach, so that intravenous therapy has little advantage unless the patient is vomiting or malabsorbing. Metabolism of the drug is decreased in hypothyroidism. Stable plasma levels are usually reached after 3-4 days where renal function is normal and after 7 days where renal impairment exists. Toxicity may be reversed with antibodies but unfortunately these are not widely available. The marginal inotropic effects of digoxin may exacerbate outflow obstruction in hypertrophic cardiomyopathy.

PATIENT 13

Answers are on pages 71–73

HISTORY

A 44 year old man is discovered collapsed at home by his diabetic wife. He has never been ill in his life before. His father however died aged 52 after a myocardial infarction and his older brother who suffers from angina pectoris is currently awaiting coronary artery bypass graft surgery. The patient is a heavy (40/day) smoker. He was made redundant 3 months previously and has since been unable to secure employment.

EXAMINATION

In the accident and emergency department he is satisfactorily self-ventilating but is unresponsive to painful stimuli: pupils are of normal size and direct and consensual light reflexes are normal: all limbs are flaccid: plantar response is equivocal on both sides. Crepitations are noted in both lungs. BP 160/100 mmHg in the right arm. Pulse 100/minute regular. Heart sounds pure. No murmurs.

ECG: sinus tachycardia; T inversion in Vl-V6.

QUESTIONS

1. What is the differential diagnosis?

2. What investigations do you consider important?

Multiple choice questions

3. Complications of external cardiac massage include:

(a) haemothorax

(b) left ventricular rupture

(c) aortic rupture

(d) laceration of spleen

(e) acute tricuspid regurgitation

4. Acute pulmonary oedema may follow:

(a) inhalation of Belair

(b) fibreoptic bronchoscopy

(c) rapid ascent to high altitude

(d) elective cardioversion

(e) aspiration of gastric contents

5. In patients with a clinical diagnosis of myocardial infarction:

(a) the presence of left bundle branch block prevents an ECG diagnosis of myocardial infarction

(b) deep symmetrical T wave inversion in Vl and V2 is likely if a true posterior infarct is present

(c) Q waves in a patient with right bundle branch block must be disregarded

(d) a change in axis is usually unimportant

(e) classical ECG changes of transmural infarction never return to normal.

6. Primary pulmonary hypertension:

(a) may be associated with ingestion of the oral contraceptive pill

(b) is often accompanied by Raynaud's phenomenon

(c) is frequently complicated by exertional syncope

(d) may only be firmly diagnosed after pulmonary angiography, but cardiac catheterisation is hazardous and potentially lethal

(e) may follow ingestion of appetite suppressant drugs

7. Parenteral morphine

(a) may precipitate acute renal failure

(b) has vasodilator action in pulmonary oedema

(c) should be administered as a rapid intravenous bolus

(d) is contraindicated in the Wolff-Parkinson-White syndrome

(e) is absolutely contraindicated in patients with chronic bronchitis and emphysema

ANSWERS AND DISCUSSION

PATIENT 13

1. Differential diagnosis
   (a) subendocardial myocardial infarction (note family history).
   (b) primary ventricular fibrillation with cerebral hypoxia, the arrhythmia having resolved by the time of presentation.
   (c) subarachnoid haemorrhage with neurogenic pulmonary oedema.
   (d) depression leading to overdose of insulin with hypoglycaemia — note availability of insulin.

2. Important investigations include
    (a) plasma glucose, urea and electrolytes (especially potassium)
    (b) ECG, cardiac enzymes
    (c) chest X-ray
    (d) arterial blood gases
    (e) computerised tomography brain scan ± lumbar puncture.

3. TRUE   TRUE   TRUE   TRUE   TRUE

Overvigorous external cardiac massage by medical as well as paramedical personnel may cause rupture of many cardiac structures and laceration of abdominal viscera. The true incidence of these side effects is unknown since the underlying vascular lesion may be presumed to be the cause of death.

4. FALSE   FALSE   TRUE   TRUE   TRUE

High altitude pulmonary oedema and that which occasionally follows elective cardioversion are ill understood phenomena. Inhalation of acid gastric contents (Mendelson's syndrome of obstetric practice) results in altered alveolar capillary membrane permeability with pulmonary oedema.

5. TRUE   FALSE   FALSE   FALSE   FALSE

Left bundle branch block obscures the usual transmural infarct pattern, but Q waves in V5 and V6 remain of significance, and ectopics occurring as part of the same trace may occasionally show the underlying infarct pattern. Pathological Q waves in a patient with right bundle branch block still signify infarction. T waves in VI and V2 are usually upright in a true posterior infarction. A change in axis may indicate extension of damaged myocardium, with possible change from left anterior to posterior hemiblock, and heralding complete heart block. After transmural myocardial infarction around one tenth of ECGs will be normal at 1 year.

6. TRUE   TRUE   TRUE   TRUE   TRUE

Associated factors in the development of primary pulmonary hypertension include ingestion of the oral contraceptive pill and some appetite suppressant drugs. Theories regarding the aetiology of the condition abound, but none is proven. Common symptoms include syncope and dyspnoea on exertion, praecordial chest pain, weakness, palpitation, cough and occasionally haemoptysis. Right heart failure may supervene. Raynaud's phenomenon is a not uncommon finding. Pulmonary angiography is necessary to arrive at the diagnosis, demonstrating large proximal pulmonary arteries with peripheral tapering, but patients may be too ill to tolerate the procedure.

7. TRUE   TRUE   FALSE   FALSE   FALSE

Opiate, by virtue of its vasodilator action among others, is most valuable in the treatment of pulmonary oedema, but may produce hypotension with acute or acute on chronic renal failure in susceptible patients. The drug should be administered cautiously, titrating the dose to the patient's needs. Indeed given cautiously opiate is most valuable in controlling myocardial pain in patients with airways obstruction. There is no contraindication to the use of opiate in the Wolff-Parkinson-White syndrome.

PATIENT 14

Answers are on pages 77–79

HISTORY

A 66 year old housewife is admitted for control of hypertension. She has received hypotensive drugs for 20 years but blood pressure control has only deteriorated over the past year. Previous investigation has shown a right duplex kidney with a double ureter, and renal cortical scarring suggestive of previous parenchymal infection. Other current complaints are of angina pectoris for 5 years and intermittent claudication in the left leg for 2 years. Drugs on admission consist of frusemide 80 mg b.d., propranolol 320 mg b.d. and methyldopa 500 mg t.i.d.

EXAMINATION

BP 280/146 mmHg, pulse 66/min regular. Sclerosed radial arteries. Optic fundi — arteriovenous nipping, but no haemorrhages or exudates. Bilateral basal crepitations. Normal abdominal examination. No neurological deficit.

INITIAL INVESTIGATIONS

Haemoglobin 10.6 g/dl. ESR 62 mm in one hour. Haematrocrit 32% MCV 79 fl. MCH 32 pg. MCHC 33 g/dl. Creatinine clearance 20 ml/min. 2.4 g/24 hours of urinary protein. Serum electrolytes: sodium 136 mmol/l, potassium 3.5 mmol/l, bicarbonate 21 mmol/l, urea 25 mmol/l, creatinine 270 μmol/l.

MANAGEMENT

BP control (160/90 mmHg) is achieved with captopril 25 mg t.i.d. and frusemide 80 mg b.d., but on this regimen the serum creatinine concentration rises to 650 μmol/l over 3 days. Captopril is withdrawn, and over 4 days the serum creatinine falls to 300 μmol/l but the BP rises to 210/120 mmHg. Reintroduction of a more modest dose of captopril produces a BP of 180/100 mmHg but a serum creatinine of 490 μmol/l.

QUESTIONS

1. What possible explanations can you offer for the patient's proteinuria?

2. What possible explanations can you offer for her anaemia?

3. What explanation can you offer for the changes in renal function with treatment?

4. What further investigations, if any, are indicated?

Multiple choice questions

5. Oral converting enzyme inhibitor (captopril):

(a) *inhibits the enzyme responsible for the conversion of angiotensin II to breakdown products*

(b) *produces the nephrotic syndrome in the majority of cases*

(c) *may precipitate hyperkalaemic crises*

(d) *is highly effective on its own in the treatment of intractable hypertension*

(e) *bears significant chemical similarities to penicillamine.*

6. When oral converting enzyme inhibitor is administered to a patient with renal artery stenosis:

(a) *there may be a precipitate fall in blood pressure with the first dose*

(b) *the full hypotensive effect of the maximal recommended dose will be achieved within a few days*

(c) *the dose need not be reduced in the presence of impaired renal function*

(d) *mechanisms other than alterations in the renin — angiotensin system may be responsible for the blood pressure reduction*

(e) *it is important to monitor the full blood count monthly*

7. Hypertension may be caused by renal artery stenosis. Renal artery stenosis in turn may be caused by:

(a) *trauma*

(b) *phaeochromocytoma*

(c) *gravid uterus*

(d) *crura of the diaphragm*

(e) *psoas abscess.*

8. In a hypertensive patient with chronic renal failure the following are common symptoms:

(a) *pruritis*

(b) *paraesthesiae*

(c) *palpitation*

(d) *diarrhoea*

(e) *swollen ankles.*

9. Renal ischaemia may cause:

(a) *crescent formation in Bowman's capsule*

(b) *hypertrophy of the juxtaglomerular apparatus*

(c) *cortical scarring*

(d) *acute tubular necrosis*

(e) *hydronephrosis*

ANSWERS AND DISCUSSION

PATIENT 14

1. Proteinuria could be due to hypertensive renal damage or to underlying renal disease which has caused the hypertension e.g. chronic glomerulonephritis or pyelonephritis or even renal artery stenosis. It is important to note that proteinuria has antedated the use of captopril.

2. The secondary anaemia of chronic renal failure is the likeliest cause, although haemolytic anaemia secondary to ingestion of methyldopa has not been excluded on the available information.

3. In this patient the elevated blood pressure appears to be necessary for adequate renal perfusion. Good hypotensive control has produced an unusual form of prerenal renal failure, suggestive of bilateral renal artery disease with, typically, a renal artery occlusion on one side and a tight stenosis on the other.

4. Renal arteriography and renal vein sampling are indicated if not from the point of view of attempting to control blood pressure surgically (since hypertension has been present for many years), though even at this late stage an improvement in control may be achieved, then certainly from the point of view of preserving or improving renal function. Although open surgery would usually be contraindicated in a patient of this age the alternative to surgery may be fatal renal failure; the recent development of percutaneous transluminal angioplasty provides an alternative approach.

5. FALSE   FALSE   TRUE   FALSE   TRUE

Captopril inhibits the enzyme responsible for converting the relatively inactive decapeptide angiotensin I to the potent pressor octapeptide angiotensin II. It is usually effective on its own in the treatment of renal artery stenosis, and in combination with loop diuretics in the management of intractable hypertension. It bears certain chemical similarities to penicillamine (particularly its sulphydryl group) and shares many side effects including skin rashes and taste disturbance (common side effects) and a membraneous glomerulopathy and blood dyscrasias (rarely). Since plasma aldosterone levels fall markedly with captopril therapy a rise in serum potassium of around 1 mmol/l is not uncommon, and in patients with underlying renal impairment may precipitate hyperkalaemia.

6. TRUE   FALSE   FALSE   TRUE   FALSE

Where the arterial pressure is dependent on a high circulating angiotensin II level as may be the case in renal artery stenosis or in conditions of sodium depletion the first dose of captopril may produce a precipitate fall in blood pressure that may require to be remedied with an intravenous infusion of angiotensin or of hypernormal saline. The full hypotensive effect of captopril may not be seen for several weeks in patients with renal artery stenosis, perhaps due to reversal of the slow pressor effects of angiotensin II though other actions mediated through the kinin and prostaglandin systems may play a part. In the presence of renal failure the dose of captopril should be reduced; there is evidence that the renal side effects of the drug are largely related to the higher dosage regimens in patients with impaired renal function. Blood dyscrasias occur usually early in the course of treatment if at all but are rare.

7. TRUE   TRUE   FALSE   TRUE   FALSE

Atheroma and fibromuscular hyperplasia with or without thrombosis are the commonest causes of renal artery stenosis, but external pressure on the renal arteries from tumours, cysts, diaphragmatic crura or sympathetic chains are recognized and constitute a Goldblatt 2-kidney model of experimental hypertension. Blunt abdominal trauma or deceleration injuries by disrupting the intima of the renal artery may lead to renal artery thrombosis. The gravid uterus and psoas abscess are not known to cause renal artery stenosis, though some workers have forwarded a hypothesis that stretching of the renal arteries by the uterus during pregnancy may contribute to the development of the fibromuscular hyperplasia.

8. TRUE   TRUE   FALSE   FALSE   TRUE

In chronic renal failure whether secondary to hypertensive damage or not, pruritus (due to accumulation of nitrogenous breakdown products in the skin) paraesthesiae (due to secondary hyperparathyroidism) and swollen ankles (due to hypoproteinaemia/proteinuria or to the secondary anaemia of renal failure) are common symptoms. Palpitations and diarrhoea may occur for a variety of reasons but are not common.

9. FALSE   TRUE   TRUE   TRUE   TRUE

Distal to a renal artery stenosis hypertrophy of the juxtaglomerular apparatus is to be expected, in keeping with a high concentration of renin in renal venous blood — before assays for renin were readily available renal biopsy and assessment of the degree of hypertrophy of this sort was one test used to assess surgical prognosis. Fibrosis and scarring may occur because of ischaemic damage distal to disease of small as well as large renal arteries. Acute tubular necrosis may be found in a kidney with an occluded main renal artery. Hydronephrosis may be caused by large periureteric collaterals though the abnormality is more often apparent radiologically than is the case clinically. Crescent formation is not a feature of ischaemia.

PATIENT 15

Answers are on pages 82–84

HISTORY

A 36 year old mother of two children, aged 10 and 6 years, presents to the medical outpatient clinic with a 3 month history of retrosternal discomfort on exertion, radiating to the left shoulder, relieved by rest, and lasting 5 minutes on each occasion. Previous medical histroy includes appendicectomy (age 10), frequent urinary tract infections in childhood, and migraine for 5 years.

EXAMINATION

Examination reveals no abnormality.
　　Chest X-ray and ECG are normal.

QUESTIONS

1. What additional clinical information would you find helpful?

2. Which five blood tests would be most helpful?

3. Are further investigations indicated, and if so which?

Multiple choice questions

4. With regard to the epidemiology of coronary artery disease which of the following statements is/are true?

(a) *The incidence of myocardial infarction among male Scots has doubled between the mid 19th and mid 20th centuries.*

(b) *The fall in the death rate from coronary heart disease in the USA during the 1970s was due to a change to a diet rich in polyunsaturated fats.*

(c) *The death rate from coronary heart disease is low in Japan.*

(d) *The Minnesota code is a useful means of coding symptoms of coronary heart disease.*

(e) *The best indicator of future death from myocardial infarction is the presence of coronary heart disease itself.*

5. Which of these statements is/are true?

(a) *Plasma concentrations of high density lipoproteins have been positively correlated with exercise.*

(b) *Frederickson Type IIA hyperlipoproteinaemia (hypercholesterolaemia) may be produced by diabetes mellitus.*

(c) *Alcohol excess and hypertriglyceridaemia are positively correlated.*

(d) *Hypertriglyceridaemia has been clearly linked with an increased risk of developing coronary heart disease.*

(e) *The benefits of lowering plasma lipids in terms of a decreased morbidity and mortality from coronary events has been clearly shown.*

6. Atherosclerosis:

(a) *affects most extensively the abdominal aorta in comparison with other blood vessels.*

(b) *has been shown to be due principally to insudation of plasma lipids through damaged endothelium*

(c) *predominantly affects medium and small-bore arteries*

CARDIOLOGY REVISION

(d) *is the longterm sequel to aortic fatty streaks in infants*

(e) *may regress following dietary manipulations.*

7. During normal pregnancy:

(a) *pulmonary vascular resistance rises*

(B) *blood volume increases by up to 50%*

(c) *maximum cardiac output is reached in the middle trimester and is maintained until full-term*

(d) *minute volume is increased*

(e) *a continuous murmur maximal in the second right intercostal space may be innocent.*

8. During pregnancy:

(a) *valvotomy is contraindicated for patients with mitral stenosis*

(b) *endocarditis is a concern in patients with atrial septal defect*

(c) *antibiotic prophylaxis is indicated throughout the third trimester in patients with ventricular septal defect*

(d) *fatal cardiomyopathy may develop in the third trimester*

(e) *patients with congenital heart block suffer from frequent syncopal episodes.*

ANSWERS AND DISCUSSION

PATIENT 15

1. Smoking habits
Use of the oral contraceptive pill/age at menopause/? oophorectomy

Previous blood pressure measurements
Family history of ischaemic heart disease, hypertension, hyperlipidaemia or endocrine disorder
Features of diabetes mellitus, hypothyroidism or anaemia

2. Full blood count
Urea and electrolytes
Fasting plasma glucose
Fasting cholesterol and triglycerides
Thyroxine (TSH level)

3. Exercise tolerance test
Echocardiogram to confirm normality of valves
Cardiac catheterization with coronary angiography

4. FALSE   FALSE   TRUE   FALSE   TRUE

Non-fatal acute myocardial infarction only began to be recognized as an uncommon disease entity at the beginning of the 20th century. The incidence of fatal coronary disease has fallen recently in the USA but though changes in dietary and exercise habits are probably contributory, the explanation is not known. In Japan the death rate has remained low. The best prognostic index of fatal infarction to come is indeed present coronary artery disease. The Minnesota code is used for ECG analysis in epidemiological studies.

5. TRUE   FALSE   TRUE   FALSE   FALSE

The correlation between exercise and apparently 'protective' high density lipoproteins is an interesting one. Diabetes mellitus, and alcoholism, are associated with hypertriglyceridaemia but this hyperlipidaemia does not have a clear association with an increased risk of coronary heart disease. Further, the benefits of lowering cholesterol (for which clear evidence of an association with coronary artery disease exists) have not been clearly demonstrated. Note also that the evidence for benefit of reducing elevated arterial pressure in terms of decreased morbidity and mortality from coronary artery disease is scanty.

6. TRUE FALSE FALSE FALSE TRUE

Atherosclerosis principally affects large and medium sized arteries, involvement of the abdominal aorta being most extensive. The main theories of the pathogenesis of atherosclerosis revolve round 'insudation' or 'encrustation': the true explanation may be a balance of the two effects. The role of the fatty streak in the development of atherosclerosis has come under critical review recently and it is by no means clear if it has a direct relationship to atheroma formation. By angiography atheromatous plaques may be observed to regress, and this may occur contemporaneously with manipulation in dietary lipids — a uniform response does not occur, however, and the relationship remains to be proven in large series.

7. FALSE TRUE TRUE TRUE TRUE

In normal pregnancy physiological alterations include increased cardiac output maximal from the middle trimester onwards, increased stroke volume, heart rate, blood volume, minute ventilation, and oxygen consumption, plus decreased blood pressure, systemic and pulmonary vascular resistance, and airway resistance. A continuous murmur maximal in the second right interspace is probably that of a mammary souffle, best heard with the patient flat, or of a venous hum.

8. FALSE FALSE FALSE TRUE FALSE

Endocarditis is rarely provoked by pregnancy, and antibiotic prophylaxis during the third trimester is not indicated. Patients with congenital heart block do well, and symptoms are unusual. Closed mitral valvotomy may prove necessary and lifesaving during pregnancy. A form of idiopathic congestive cardiomyopathy is well recognized in the last trimester or postpartum period, and may be rapidly fatal; where the syndrome resolves it is likely to recur in a subsequent pregnancy.

PATIENT 16

Answers are on pages 88–90

HISTORY

A 66 year old widow, who has suffered no significant past illnesses, is rushed to the accident department following a 2 minute dizzy spell which occurred during a visit to her local grocer's shop. She described a feeling of 'lightheadedness' and apprehension with no loss of awareness of her surroundings, no vertigo, no features of epilepsy and no chest pain or palpitation. She is a non-smoker, but admits to drinking two glasses of sherry each day.

EXAMINATION

Blood pressure 130/70 mmHg in the right arm, lying; pulse 64/min, regular; heart sounds pure; no murmurs. No neurological deficit.
Chest X-ray and ECG are normal.

MANAGEMENT

The patient is subsequently discharged home.
8 hours later the patient is 'crashed' into casualty following a collapse at home. On this occasion she is clammy, cold

and sweating profusely; blood pressure 80 mmHg systolic by palpation of the radial pulse; pulse 130/minute, weak but regular; a grade 3/6 systolic murmur is audible over the whole praecordium. There are widespread crepitations.

QUESTIONS

1. What is the differential diagnosis on the first assessment?

2. What is the differential diagnosis on the second assessment?

3. Which investigations are required to clarify the diagnosis?

4. How would you manage this patient?

Multiple choice questions

5. The frequency of ventricular extrasystoles is associated with:

(a) *the size of a myocardial infarction*

(b) *the poverty of left ventricular function after myocardial infarction*

(c) *the development of premature coronary heart disease in otherwise healthy individuals*

(d) *exercise in healthy individuals*

(e) *excessive plasma levels of quadricyclic drugs*

6. The occurrence of the following features in a patient with acute myocardial infarction signifies a poor prognosis:

(a) *hypertension*

(b) *cardiomegaly*

(c) *pericarditis*

(d) *second degree atrioventricular block in an inferior myocardial infarction*

(e) *atrial fibrillation in anterior infarction.*

7. Prinzmetal (variant) angina:

(a) *may be made worse by treatment with beta-blockers*

(b) *is associated with an increased incidence of sudden death*

(c) *may be precipitated by phentolamine*

(d) *is rarely associated with atherosclerosis of the coronary arteries*

(e) *may be associated with the transient appearance of Q waves on the ECG*

8. Following coronary artery bypass graft surgery:

(a) *mortality from coronary heart disease is decreased in patients with single, double and triple vessel disease*

(b) *in patients with unstable angina only a small minority of patients fail to experience substantial or complete relief from symptoms*

(c) *ankle oedema secondary to congestive cardiac failure is a common problem*

(d) *heavy goods vehicle licences are generally withdrawn*

(e) *long-term psychiatric illness is common.*

9. Radionuclide ventriculography:

(a) *is useful in determining alterations in ejection fraction with exercise*

(b) *results are compromised by frequent ventricular ectopics.*

(c) *commonly employs ^{131}I-albumin as the radiopharmaceutical*

(d) *involves radiation to the patient greater than that from a standard intravenous urogram*

(e) *may be used to predict patients at high risk of suffering heart failure and sudden death in the year after a first myocardial infarction.*

ANSWERS AND DISCUSSION

PATIENT 16

1. Vasovagal episode
   Vertebrobasilar insufficiency
   Epileptic fit
   Hypoglycaemia
   Arrhythmia
   'Silent' myocardial infarction

2. Myocardial infarction complicated by a ruptured ventricular septum or by a ruptured papillary muscle with mitral regurgitation.

3. ECG, chest X–ray, echocardiogram, cardiac catheterization.

4. Surgery to repair the ventricular septum is best delayed until the patient is fitter — the operative mortality in the acute phase is extremely high. Likewise mitral valve replacement should be delayed for at least a week after myocardial infarction if the clinical state of the patient allows this.

5. TRUE TRUE FALSE FALSE TRUE

The frequency of ventricular ectopics has been correlated with the size of myocardial infarction and poor left ventricular function during recovery from myocardial infarction. Ventricular ectopics occur sporadically in healthy young people, the frequency increases with age, and do not in their own right confer a poor prognosis in otherwise healthy people. Excessive plasma levels of tricyclic or quadricyclic antidepressant drugs commonly precipitate ventricular ectopics and these may herald more sinister arrhythmias.

6. FALSE TRUE FALSE FALSE TRUE

Hypertension may contribute to cardiac rupture after infarction, but rarely signifies a poor prognosis. Pericarditis is common and often transient while second degree block in inferior myocardial infarction is often a transient phenomenon with rapid spontaneous recovery. Atrial fibrillation, cardiomegaly, persistent sinus tachycardia, hypotension and cardiac failure, late ventricular arrhythmias, high degrees of atrioventricular block in anterior myocardial infarction and new bundle branch block are all associated with an adverse prognosis.

7. TRUE TRUE FALSE FALSE TRUE

Prinzmetal angina is episodic and usually short-lived, unrelated to exercise, accompanied by ST segment elevation and even Q wave development, which return to normal with pain relief, is associated with ventricular tachyarrhythmias, myocardial infarction and sudden death, and is thought to be due to spasm of a coronary artery with a normal underlying vessel or with an underlying fixed stenosis. The syndrome may be largely mediated by alpha-adrenergic fibres, such that beta-blockers may be to the patient's detriment. Nifedipine and nitrates are most helpful in the medical management while beta-blockers often *may* be helpful.

8. FALSE TRUE FALSE TRUE FALSE

Mortality is definitely improved for patients with left main stem disease and marginally for patients with triple vessel disease; the quality of life is greatly improved in all groups. Symptomatically coronary artery bypass graft surgery is very successful in patients with unstable angina. Following such surgery HGV licences are withdrawn. Ankle oedema is usually the result of removal of the long saphenous system for grafts. Psychiatric disturbances in the immediate postoperative period are not uncommon, but longterm sequellae are rare.

9. TRUE TRUE FALSE FALSE TRUE

Pertechnetate (^{99m}Tc) is the radiopharmaceutical of choice for radionuclide ventriculography, the radiation dose to the patient being small (around 250 millirads), and the investigation yields useful information on ejection fraction at rest and with exercise. Frequent ventricular ectopics compromise these measurements. Ejection fraction measured by this technique has proved accurate in predicting which patients will develop heart failure, recurrent arrhythmia and sudden death in the year after a first myocardial infarction.

PATIENT 17

Answers are on pages 93–96

HISTORY

A 43 year old housewife who has been an insulin-dependent diabetic for 16 years presents with a 1 week history of malaise, drowsiness and visual blurring. For 2 weeks she has experienced occipital headaches and has developed nocturia twice nightly. 2 weeks previously she experienced transient left loin pain, but this resolved within 24 hours. She is a 30/day cigarette smoker, and in addition takes pizotifen for migraine prophylaxis.

EXAMINATION

On examination she is thin and dehydrated. BP 206/130 mmHg lying. Pulse 90/min regular. Optic fundi — bilateral flame shaped haemorrhages and hard exudates with blurring of the left optic disc. Abdominal examination unremarkable.

INITIAL INVESTIGATIONS

Serum electrolyte concentrations: sodium 126 mmol/l, potassium 2.5 mmol/l, bicarbonate 20 mmol/l, urea 26 mmol/l. Creatinine clearance 26 ml/min. Urinalysis: 2% glucose, 1 + ketones. Plasma glucose 32 mmol/l.

QUESTIONS

1. What is the differential diagnosis?

2. Name the single test most likely to identify the cause of the hypertension.

3. How would you manage this patient?

Multiple choice questions

4. Secondary hyperaldosteronism is a common finding in:

(a) *congestive cardiac failure*

(b) *ascites*

(c) *excess liquorice ingestion*

(d) *polycystic kidney disease*

(e) *nephrotic syndrome.*

5. Cigarette smoking is significantly commoner in patients suffering from the following conditions compared with those suffering from benign essential hypertension:

(a) *phaeochromocytoma*

(b) *renal artery stenosis*

(c) *malignant phase hypertension*

(d) *Conn's syndrome*

(e) *Cushing's syndrome.*

6. The following drugs would be relatively contraindicated in the management of a hypertensive 60 year old diabetic (treated with chlorpropamide and diet) who 2 weeks previously had suffered a right sided stroke with mild expressive dysphasia:

(a) *hydrallazine*

(b) *bendrofluazide*

(c) *methylodopa*

(d) *propranolol*

(e) *prazosin.*

7. Creatinine clearance of 50 ml/min based on a 24 hour urine save in a patient with normal serum urea and creatinine concentrations:

(a) *probably indicates an incomplete urine collection*

(b) *may be normal in a bilateral amputee*

(c) *indicates incipient renal failure*

(d) *suggests that the patient is on oral antituberculous drugs*

(e) *may be normal in a 10 year old child.*

8. The following conditions should be considered when a hypertensive patient is admitted with delusions:

(a) *acute intermittent porphyria*

(b) *salicylate poisoing*

(c) *systemic lupus erythematosus*

(d) *malignant phase hypertension*

(e) *hydronephrosis.*

ANSWERS AND DISCUSSION

PATIENT 17

1. The features of malignant phase hypertension following a history suggestive of left renal infarction with concomitant hyponatraemia and hypokalaemia are consistent with a diagnosis of the hyponatraemic hypertensive syndrome. In this syndrome the rapid onset of severe hypertension in the presence of one relatively normal kidney results in a pressure natriuresis in the normal kidney with the ensuing biochemical picture described above.

This patient has also experienced loss of diabetic control with ketoacidosis. The serum bicarbonate level of 20 mmol/l reflects a balance between diabetic metabolic acidosis and hypokalaemic alkalosis.

2. Renal arteriography.

3. Initial management should be directed at controlling her diabetes with intravenous saline, potassium and insulin, and at controlling her blood pressure. In view of the likelihood of left renal artery occlusion and in the presence of marked hyponatraemia this patient's plasma renin and angiotensin II concentrations are likely to be markedly elevated. A small dose of captropril (oral converting enzyme inhibitor) is the most logical hypotensive drug in these circumstances but may produce a profound fall in blood pressure. Angiotensin II (Hypertensin, Ciba) or hypernormal saline should be available to reverse this hypotension should it occur.

On the basis of further investigation either reconstructive renal artery surgery or left nephrectomy may cure this patient's hypertension, but should be performed as a semi-elective or elective procedure.

4. TRUE   TRUE   FALSE   FALSE   TRUE

In secondary hyperaldosteronism the renin-angiotensin-aldosterone axis has been stimulated throughout by a trigger such as hyponatraemia, reduced renal plasma flow, hypotension and many others. Hyponatraemia may be a feature of congestive cardiac failure, ascites and the nephrotic syndrome, though other triggers may be present, and often the therapy for these conditions, including powerful diuretics, may exacerbate the hyponatraemia and the hyperaldosteronism. Spironolactone in these circumstances is a useful drug. Patients ingesting an excess of liquorice, with its mineralocorticoid constituent, tend to have low plasma aldosterone levels. Polycystic kidney disease does not usually disturb the renin angiotensin aldosterone system except in the very late stages of the disease.

5. FALSE   TRUE   TRUE   FALSE   FALSE

Patients with phaeochromocytoma or adrenal cortical adenoma with autonomous hypersecretion of mineralocorticoids or glucocorticoids suffer from neoplasia for which no firm association has been established with cigarette smoking. On the other hand there is strong evidence that 80–90% of patient with malignant phase hypertension smoke and when compared with age sex and blood pressure matched patients without malignant phase hypertension (around 50% smoked) the difference is highly significant statistically; the explanation of this phenomenon is uncertain. Likewise there is a high incidence of cigarette smoking among patients with all forms of renal artery stenosis, both atheromatous and fibromuscular hyperplasia; a plausible explanation revolves round the thrombogenic effects of smoking on already diseased vessels, worsening the stenosis and leading to clinical presentation.

6. FALSE   TRUE   TRUE   TRUE   TRUE

This sort of patient is difficult to treat since many contraindications to particular drugs exist. Thiazide diuretics may produce a further elevation in plasma glucose. Methyldopa by producing somnolence, depression and even stupor in high dosage would be undesirable in a patient who already has cause to be depressed and in whom any alteration of conscious level would be difficult to interpret. Propranolol among other possible side effects would mask the signs and symptoms of hypoglycaemia. Prazosin by producing unpredictable collapse is relatively contraindicated though introduced under inpatient conditions it may be safe. Hydrallazine has no specific contraindications but is unsuitable administered on its own. It may be necessary to prescribe a regimen with potential side effects, realizing what these are likely to be and accepting that several combinations may have to be tried and abandoned before the ideal therapy is found.

7. TRUE   FALSE   FALSE   FALSE   FALSE

Creatinine clearance is calculated from the formula UV/P where U is the urinary concentration of creatinine in a timed collection, V is the volume of urine in that time, and P is the plasma concentration of creatinine at a representative point during that time. The clearance will thus be falsely low if V is low i.e. incomplete urine collection. The levels of urinary and plasma creatinine depend on the muscle bulk of the patient but are proportionately reduced in a child whose muscle bulk has yet largely to develop or in a patient in whom a significant proportion has been amputated, such that creatinine clearance remains normal. A reduced clearance does not indicate incipient renal failure where plasma urea and creatinine concentration are normal. The comment on antituberculous therapy is irrelevant.

8. TRUE   FALSE   TRUE   TRUE   FALSE

Porphyria, systemic lupus erythematosus, phaeochromocytoma and Cushing's syndrome may be causes of a primary psychiatric presentation in patients who are then found to be hypertensive. In malignant phase hypertension with encephalopathy psychiatric symptoms may be clamant. Salicylate poisoning and hydronephrosis do not produce such symptoms.

PATIENT 18

Answers are on pages 99–101

HISTORY

A 40 year old engineer is transferred urgently to the coronary care unit from a general surgical ward, complaining of severe retrosternal discomfort which he has experienced on recovering consciousness after elective right inguinal herniorrhaphy. He smokes 30 cigarettes daily and his father died age 56 following a myocardial infarction. However he has never experienced symptoms of ischaemic heart disease himself, and his ECG preoperatively was normal. He has never been in hospital before.

EXAMINATION

On examination he is normal. BP 130/80 mmHg in the right arm, lying. Pulse 80/min, regular. Heart sounds pure. No evidence of cardiac failure. Respiratory examination normal.
Repeat ECG — normal.

QUESTIONS

1. What is the differential diagnosis?

2. What treatment should you give?

Multiple choice questions

3. Patients with acute pulmonary embolism may present with:

(a) systemic hypotension

(b) exertional dyspnoea

(c) pulmonary oedema

(d) abdominal pain

(e) recurrent pleurisy.

4. Which of the following statements is/are true?

(a) T wave inversion in leads V4-V6 may suggest pulmonary embolism in an acutely ill patient

(b) Abnormal perfusion scans are diagnostic of pulmonary embolism

(c) Return to normal of abnormal perfusion scans is powerful evidence of resolving pulmonary infarction.

(d) Thrombolytic therapy speeds the resolution of pulmonary embolism in comparison with heparin therapy.

(e) Pulmonary angiography though helpful is not a definitive investigation in suspected pulmonary embolism.

5. Which of the following drugs may cause myocardial damage?

(a) Emetine.

(b) Paracetamol.

(c) Adriamycin.

(d) Baclofen.

(e) Lithium carbonate.

6. Which of the following statements is/are true?

(a) Torsade de pointes (paroxysmal ventricular fibrillation) during quinidine therapy most often occurs in patients with prolonged QT intervals before treatment.

(b) *Following excessive beta-blockade in the treatment of supraventricular tachycardia, glucagon may overcome the adverse effects.*
(c) *Phenytoin and procainamide have indistinguishable effects on the action potential.*
(d) *Reducing plasma potassium is an important facet of the treatment of quinidine toxicity.*
(e) *Quinidine acts primarily by prolonging the effective refractory period of the action potential.*

7. Which of the following statements regarding sympathomimetic agents is/are true?
(a) *Dopamine releases noradrenaline from the heart.*
(b) *Salbutamol exerts beneficial effects in cardiac failure by stimulation of peripheral beta receptors.*
(c) *Dobutamine is less arrhythmogenic than isoprenaline.*
(d) *Dobutamine is a synthetic analogue of noradrenaline.*
(e) *Dopamine in high doses causes vasoconstriction through stimulation of $beta_1$ receptors.*

ANSWERS AND DISCUSSION

PATIENT 18

1. Differential diagnosis
    (a) Acute myocardial infarction — the ECG changes have not yet developed.
    (b) Pulmonary embolism — unduly early, but nevertheless a possible problem.

(c) Pneumothorax complicating anaesthesia.
(d) Inadequately reversed suxamethonium effect. Suxamethonium (succinylcholine) is a depolarizing neuromuscular blocking agent which is short acting and often used in anaesthesia. The action of the drug is prolonged over 3–4 minutes in patients with low plasma levels of pseudocholinesterase. This may be a genetically determined deficiency or the result of anaemia, thyrotoxicosis, electrolyte imbalance or severe liver disease. In this patient pseudocholinesterase deficiency could have led to cramping chest discomfort, reversible with the use of additional neostigmine (question 2).

3. TRUE   TRUE   FALSE   TRUE   TRUE

Acute pulmonary embolism may present with pleuritic chest pain, dyspnoea, apprehension, cough, haemoptysis, sweating, or acute syncope. Furthermore, atypical presentations may occur, notably abdominal pain and bronchospasm mimicking a surgical abdomen and asthma respectively.

4. FALSE   FALSE   TRUE   TRUE   FALSE

ECG changes which characteristicaly occur are the S1 Q3 T3 pattern, P pulmonale and acute right heart strain with right bundle branch block, complete or incomplete, right axis deviation, and T inversion in right heart leads; also arrhythmias particularly ventricular ectopics or less commonly atrial fibrillation may occur. Perfusion scan abnormalities may be caused by many pathologies including emphysema, but resolution of wedge-shaped areas of hypoperfusion is persuasive evidence of pulmonary infarction. Streptokinase/urokinase speeds lysis of pulmonary emboli, but since the treatment involves hazards in its own right it is usually reserved for severely ill patients who do not warrant surgical intervention. Pulmonary angiography is the most specific test available in the diagnosis of pulmonary embolism.

5. TRUE   TRUE   TRUE   FALSE   TRUE

Cardiotoxicity is an important potential side effect of many agents with widely different modes of action. Phenothiazines may cause arrhythmias; emetine, largely outmoded now in the treatment of amoebiasis, may produce a cardiomyopathy which usually reverses on withdrawal of the drug; lithium in toxic doses produces arrhythmias in a flabby dilated heart but minor ECG changes are common in asymptomatic patients; catecholamines in high dosage may cause myocarditis; paracetamol overdose though causing predominant hepatic and renal effects also produces fatty degeneration and focal myocardial necrosis; adriamycin, daunorubicin and cyclophosphamide may all produce cardiomyopathy.

6. TRUE TRUE FALSE TRUE FALSE

Quinidine is the archetypal Class I antiarrhythmic, acting principally on the fast sodium channels to produce membrane stabilization. Toxic side effects are not uncommon and include paroxysmal ventricular fibrillation, particularly if there is prolongation of the QT interval pretreatment. Normal serum potassium levels are necessary for quinidine to work properly — iatrogenic hypokalaemia will therefore reduce toxic effects; acidification of urine also encourages excretion of the drug. Procainamide has very similar properties (Class IA) to quinidine, whereas phenytoin like lignocaine (Class IB) has clearly distinguishable electrophysiological properties. Since glucagon acts at a different myocardial cell membrane receptor from beta-blocking drugs it may circumvent toxic beta-blocker effects.

7. TRUE TRUE TRUE FALSE FALSE

Dopamine is a physiological precursor of noradrenaline, but also releases noradrenaline from the heart. In high dosage dopamine vasoconstricts peripherally, through stimulation of alpha receptors. Dobutamine is a synthetic analogue of dopamine, does not release noradrenaline directly from the heart and is less arrhythmogenic than isoprenaline. Salbutamol is a relatively selective beta$_2$ agonist whose probable main action is to cause peripheral vasodilation, though a positive inotropic effect may contribute to its action.

PATIENT 19

Answers are on pages 105–107

HISTORY

A 64 year old dentist who has suffered from angina pectoris for 7 years is admitted to the coronary care unit during the night following 3 hours of intense unremitting chest pain with heaviness and paraesthesia of the left arm, nausea and vomiting. Opiate administered by his general practitioner had partially relieved the discomfort. The patient's usual medication consists of metoprolol 50 mg b.d., sublingual glyceryl trinitrate and a calcium antagonist. The patient has not smoked for 10 years. In childhood he underwent appendicectomy, and 15 years previously he underwent partial gastrectomy for a bleeding gastric ulcer.

EXAMINATION

On admission the patient is pale, clammy, cool and confused. Pupils bilaterally constricted. Tendon reflexes in legs diminished but right jerks brisker than left. Plantars equivocal bilaterally. Blood pressure 108/60 mmHg in the right arm, lying. Pulse 100/minute regular but small volume. Third and fourth heart sounds present. No murmurs. JVP +8 cm. No peripheral oedema. No crepitations.

ECG — sinus tachycardia; PR = 0.24 sec, right bundle branch block.

Chest X-ray — within normal limits.

Next morning blood pressure is 96/62 mmHg and the patient has not passed urine since admission. A catheter is passed, 220 ml urine obtained, but over the next two hours 12 ml of urine is collected.

QUESTIONS

1. What are the possible explanations of the neurological findings on admission?

2. What is the differential diagnosis of the cardiac complaint?

3. What investigations are indicated?

4. Following intravenous frusemide (40 mg) the patient passes 50 ml urine in 1 hour, but his systolic pressure falls to 70 mmHg. What is the diagnosis, and how would you manage the problem?

Multiple choice questions

5. Characteristic physical signs of acute cardiac tamponade include:

(a) *bradycardia*

(b) *low pulse pressure*

(c) *arterial pressure which falls by 10 mmHg or more during expiration*

(d) *friction rub*

(e) *hepatic enlargement*

6. The site of conduction delay is usually distal to the atrioventricular node in:

(a) *first degree A-V block*

(b) *Wenckebach Type II block*

(c) *Mobitz Type II block*

(d) *idioventricular rhythm with retrograde conduction to the atria*

(e) *nodal rhythm with the P wave following the QRS complex*

7. The following have been used to good effect in the management of intractable cardiac failure:

(a) *captopril*

(b) *minoxidil*

(c) *nifedipine*

(d) *methyldopa*

(e) *phentolamine*

8. Which of the following statements about beta-blockers are true?

(a) *The dose of propranolol should be reduced in patients with the nephrotic syndrome.*

(b) *Resting pulse rate and the response to exercise is a useful guide to compliance in patients receiving acebutolol.*

(c) *Patients who experience nightmares on one beta-blocker are likely to experience the same on an alternative beta-blocker.*

(d) *The major factor in modifying the appropriate dose of labetalol is first pass liver metalolism.*

(e) *If a beta-blocker requires to be a administered to a patient with intermittent claudication then one with intrinsic sympathomimetic activity is preferable.*

9. Nitrates:

(a) *act predominantly on coronary vessels*

(b) *may be administered as an oral spray*

(c) *may intensify the murmur of mitral valve prolapse*

(d) *are contraindicated in patients with hypertrophic cardiomyopathy*

(e) *may be of value in the treatment of acute pulmonary oedema*

ANSWERS AND DISCUSSION

PATIENT 19

1. Pupillary abnormalities are much more likely to be the result of opiate, than of brain stem disease. The asymmetrical but bilaterally diminished tendon jerks may signify peripheral neuropathy: this is not uncommon with perhexilene, a calcium antagonist, though many other causes of neuropathy such as diabetes mellitus may be relevant.

2. The history is characteristic of myocardial infarction and the ECG abnormalities compatible. The differential is that of low output states complicating myocardial infarction, i.e. either left ventricular dysfunction with high filling pressure or right ventricular infarction with low left ventricular filling pressures.

3. Swan-Ganz catheterization is required to diagnose predominantly right or left ventricular dysfunction.

4. Diuretics in a right ventricular infarction further volume deplete and vasodilate the patient with even lower filling pressures, hypotension and worse renal hypoperfusion, and may be a fatal therapeutic misjudgement. Patients with right ventricular infarcts require infusion of plasma or saline until adequate left ventricular filling pressures are obtained, and this may involve litres of fluid.

5. FALSE TRUE FALSE TRUE TRUE

Characteristic signs in acute tamponade include elevated jugular venous pressure with rapid x and y descents, tachycardia, pulsus paradoxus (where arterial pressure falls by 10 mmHg or more on inspiration — this is not in fact paradoxical but an exaggeration of the normal variation in arterial pressure with respiration), low pulse pressure (less than 30 mmHg), systemic hypotension, pericardial friction rubs (since the distribution of pericardial fluid is not uniform) and quiet heart sounds.

6. FALSE   FALSE   TRUE   TRUE   FALSE

Prolongation of the PR interval, and the Wenckebach phenomenon are usually the result of ischaemia or disease in the A-V node and proximal part of the bundle of His. In Mobitz — Type II second degree A-V block QRS complexes are usually of a bundle branch block pattern and signify disease distal to the A-V node. Likewise slow idioventricular rhythms imply antegrade block below the A-V node. By definition nodal rhythms arise in the A-V node, no matter where the P wave falls in the ECG.

7. TRUE   TRUE   TRUE   FALSE   TRUE

Minoxidil, nifedipine and phentolamine all reduce afterload in patients with cardiac failure, the former two agents causing arteriolar vasodilation by effects on vascular smooth muscle cells while phentolamine vasodilates by peripheral alpha blockade and also exerts positive myocardial inotropism. Captopril is in effect a combined venodilator and arterial dilator, greatly diminishing angiotensin II formation and delaying bradykinin degradation.

8. TRUE   FALSE   FALSE   TRUE   TRUE

Propranolol is highly protein bound — the dose of the drug should therefore be reduced in hypoproteinaemic states. Acebutolol is a drug with intrinsic sympathomimetic activity, i.e. the competitive beta receptor antagonist has partial agonist activity. Thus resting pulse rate may not be unduly depressed, and this marker of compliance cannot be used. Nightmares reflect the penetration of beta-blocker into the central nervous system, an effect largely dependent on their lipid solubility. Water miscible agents such as atenolol should therefore be relatively free from these effects. First pass liver metabolism is usually considerable with labetalol, as with other lipid soluble beta-blockers. Theoretically beta-blockers with high intrinsic sympathomimetic activity should be less detrimental in patients with claudication than those without this property.

9. FALSE   TRUE   TRUE   TRUE   TRUE

Nitrates act on both coronary vessels and systemic veins and to a lesser extent systemic arteries. Nitrates cause the murmur of mitral valve prolapse to increase because left ventricular volume is reduced, while in hypertrophic cardio-myopathy the pressure gradient may increase, the murmurs intensify and the patient's symptoms deteriorate. Their acute venodilator effects make nitrates very useful in the management of pulmonary oedema. They may be administered as tablets, to be sucked, chewed, placed under the tongue, placed inside the lip, or swallowed, as an oral spray, as paste for percutaneous absorption, or as an intravenous infusion.

PATIENT 20

Answers are on pages 111–113

HISTORY

A 42 year old cashier is referred to the medical outpatient clinic for advice regarding the management of elevated blood pressure. He has a 20 year history of exertional dyspnoea and frequent episodes of purulent sputum production of several weeks' duration each. He says he was always frail as a child but recalls no specific illnesses.

EXAMINATION

On examination he is thin and sallow. He has an audible wheeze. There is increased curvature of his nail beds, but no fluctuance or loss of angle between the nail and the nailbed. Coarse crepitations are marked at both bases. BP 210/126 mmHg. JVP + 5 cm. Liver edge 3 cm below the right costal margin. Bilateral pitting ankle oedema present. Optic fundi — arteriovenous nipping, but no haemorrhages or exudates.

INITIAL INVESTIGATIONS

Haemoglobin 10.9 g/dl. White cell count 8.9×10^9/l. MCV 86 fl. MCH 34 pg MCHC 35 g/dl. ESR 60 mm in one hour. Serum electrolytes: sodium 139 mmol/1 potassium 3.6 mmol/1 urea 12.4 mmol/1, creatinine 162 μmol/1. Creatinine clearance 60 ml/min; 3 g of urinary protein per 24 hours.

QUESTIONS

1. What are the likely diagnoses and what course of events has probably occurred?

2. List 6 useful tests and your reason for performing each.

One year after treatment with methyldopa and diuretics was commenced the patient developed postural dizziness with a BP of 90/60 mmHg lying 60/40 mmHg standing, even after withdrawal of treatment. Serum electrolytes are sodium 128 mmol/1, postassium 3.9 mmol/1, urea 14.6 mmol/1.

3. (a) What problem has now developed?
(b) How would you investigate it?
(c) What management would you advise?

Multiple choice questions

4. Hypertension is a recognized finding in:

(a) *hamartoma of the lung*

(b) *subarachnoid haemorrhage*

(c) *non-metastic bronchial carcinoma*

(d) *Loeffler's syndrome (pulmonary eosinophilia)*

(e) *staphylococcal pneumonia.*

5. Thiazide diuretic therapy in patients with hypertension may be associated with:

(a) *gout*

(b) *hyporeninaemia*

(c) *postural hypotension*

(d) *low serum bicarbonate levels*

(e) *secondary polycythaemia.*

6. Postural hypotension associated with autonomic dysfunction may be accompanied by:

(a) *tachycardia on performing mental arithmetic*

(b) *profuse sweating*

(c) *nocturnal diarrhoea*

(d) *dilated pupils*

(e) *failure to raise supine blood pressure after a sudden noise.*

7. The following may be useful in the management of postural hypotension:

(a) *converting enzyme inhibitor*

(b) *fludrocortisone*

(c) *tyramine*

(d) *elastic stockings*

(e) *oral isoprenaline.*

8. Methyldopa:

(a) *acts by inhibiting peripheral alpha receptors*

(b) *may in large doses cause stupor*

(c) *may cause gynaecomastia*

(d) *requires to be given three times daily*

(e) *is associated with regression of left ventricular hypertrophy in some animals*

ANSWERS AND DISCUSSION

PATIENT 20

1. The likely diagnoses are bronchiectasis leading to amyloidosis affecting the kidney and producing hypertension. However, since hypertension in renal amyloid is relatively uncommon, essential hypertension in a patient with bronchiectasis and amyloidosis is another possible explanation.

2. Relative to the diagnosis of bronchiectasis chest X–ray, respiratory function tests, bronchography and sputum culture would all be useful tests. Renal biopsy should confirm the diagnosis of amyloid and explain the proteinuria; intravenous urography should precede biopsy. Other causes of amyloid should be excluded.

3. (a) Addison's disease secondary to adrenal amyloid (pituitary amyloid is a further possibility).
(b) Synacthen test; plasma ACTH level.
(c) Immediate — Intravenous hydrocortisone, saline
Longterm — Prednisolone ± fludrocortisone
Aggressive treatment of bronchiectasis though amyloid may now progress despite this.

4. FALSE   TRUE   TRUE   FALSE   FALSE

Hypertension may persist for several weeks after a subarachnoid haemorrhage before resolving spontaneously. Non-metastatic bronchial carcinoma by secreting ACTH may lead to Cushing's syndrome and hypertension. Hamartoma, Loeffler's syndrome and staphylococcal pneumonia are not associated with hypertension.

5. TRUE FALSE TRUE FALSE FALSE

Thiazide diuretics tend to elevate plasma uric acid levels, elevate plasma renin concentration, and elevate plasma bicarbonate levels. By producing hyponatraemia in the elderly and by shrinking plasma volume they may precipitate postural hypotension. If plasma volume is shrunk haematocrit may be raised but this acute phenomenon does not constitute secondary polycythaemia.

6. FALSE FALSE TRUE TRUE TRUE

Manifestations of autonomic dysfunction accompanying postural hypotension include an inability to increase pulse rate or to raise blood pressure under stress, impaired sweating, an inability to constrict the pupils and altered bowel habit which is more manifest at night. There are many causes of this syndrome including the Shy-Drager syndrome, diabetes mellitus, amyloidosis, and side effects of drugs such as guanethidine.

7. FALSE TRUE TRUE TRUE FALSE

Useful therapeutic manoeuvres in postural hypotension include ingestion of fludrocortisone and a high salt diet to expand plasma volume; tyramine or other indirectly acting sympathomimetic agents (cheddar cheese is a useful source of tyramine) combined with a monoamine oxidase inhibitor to augment noradrenaline concentrations at nerve endings; and mechanical support by elastic stockings. Captopril and isoprenaline are not relevant to the management of the condition.

8. FALSE TRUE TRUE FALSE TRUE

Methyldopa acts principally within the central nervous system where a product of its metabolism, alphamethylnoradrenaline, is released from adrenergic neurones and stimulates central alpha receptors, thereby reducing the sympathetic outflow from the central nervous system. In high dosage it may cause stupor which is entirely reversible. Gynaecomastia is a well recognised but not a frequent side effect. Though the custom in the past has been to prescribe methyldopa three or four times daily the drug has been shown to act for over 24 hours after a single oral dose and many would prescribe it now only twice daily. In rats administration of methyldopa has been shown to cause regression of left ventricular hypertrophy which has not been matched during similar lowering of blood pressure by other hypotensive drugs; the extension of this phenomenon to man has not been confirmed.

PATIENT 21

Answers are on pages 117–119

HISTORY

A 32 year old woman is admitted for biopsy of a left breast lump. On routine checking the surgical houseman hears a systolic murmur which he finds difficult to localize, and consequently asks for a medical opinion. On specific enquiry you find that the patient has experienced dyspnoea on climbing hills and stairs for 4 years, that she has felt light-headed on rushing for the past year with on three occasions (one of them at rest) brief loss of consciousness, and that she has experienced some left sided and retrosternal chest discomfort on rushing for 2 years.

Her past medical history is complex and includes rheumatic fever (age 4), appendicectomy (age 10), four operations for duodenal ulceration (between ages 18 and 27) and two pregnancies (at ages 19 and 26) both of which resulted in uncomplicated full term vaginal deliveries. There is a strong family history of peptic ulceration (brother, father, uncle) while the patient's father died suddenly aged 48, cause unknown. The patient smokes 20 cigarettes daily and drinks a moderate amount of alcohol. She has recently been separated from her husband and is currently living with her boyfriend who drinks too much and occasionally beats her.

QUESTIONS

1. What differential diagnosis of the patient's cardiac complaint would you consider?

GREY CASES 115

2. Of what relevance could the family history be to the cardiac complaint?

3. What physiological manoeuvres may be of value in reaching the diagnosis?

4. What noninvasive investigations, if any, are indicated?

Multiple choice questions

5. Major Duckett-Jones criteria used in the diagnosis of acute rheumatic fever include:

(a) *erythema nodosum*

(b) *subcutaneous nodules*

(c) *arthralgia*

(d) *atrioventricular block*

(e) *Huntington's chorea.*

6. Which of the following statements regarding rheumatic fever is/are true?

(a) *Absence of carditis during acute rheumatic fever ensures freedom from rheumatic valvular disease in the longterm.*

(b) *Most cardiac deaths within the first 5 years after acute rheumatic fever are due to severe mitral valve disease.*

(c) *Recurrences of acute rheumatic fever may be prevented by antibiotics.*

(d) *The chances of developing acute rheumatic fever are not increased by a previous attack.*

(e) *Restenosis of the mitral valve after closed mitral valvotomy implies recurrence of rheumatic fever with further damage to the mitral valve.*

7. Alcoholic cardiomyopathy:

(a) *may regress if alcohol consumption is stopped*

(b) *often presents with paroxysmal atrial fibrillation*

(c) is frequently associated with thromboembolic disease
(d) is often improved significantly by propranolol
(e) is accompanied by other evidence of alcohol excess — hepatic or neurological.

8. With regard to cardiac myxoma:

(a) the commonest presentation is with the symptoms and signs of mitral valve disease
(b) there is no familial association
(c) cardiac myxomas occur exclusively in the atria
(d) patients may present with cachexia
(e) some authorities believe myxoma is organized thrombus.

9. In patients with ventricular septal defect:

(a) aortic regurgitation both congenital and acquired is not an uncommon finding
(b) spontaneous closure of the defect does not alter the risk of developing infective endocarditis
(c) who also have right ventricular outflow tract obstruction relief from dyspnoea may be effected by crossing their legs
(d) as part of the tetralogy of Fallot, survival into adulthood untreated is possible because rich bronchial collaterals develop.
(d) large amplitude biphasic QRS complexes are common throughout the chest leads of the ECG.

GREY CASES 117

ANSWERS AND DISCUSSION

PATIENT 21

1. The symptoms suggest intermittent interruption of expulsion of blood from the left ventricle. This may be due to aortic stenosis, valvar, subvalvar or supravalvar, hypertrophic cardiomyopathy or atrial myxoma. Rheumatic aortic stenosis would be unusual at her age; a normal pregnancy 6 years before and anaesthesia 4 years before where presumably no murmur was heard, also go against this diagnosis. The possibility of atrial myxoma could be indicated by the one episode of loss of consciousness at rest, but in both other differential diagnoses paroxysmal tachyarrhythmias are a common cause of collapse as well as exertional syncope. In view of the patient's age and family history hypertrophic cardiomyopathy is most likely to be the correct diagnosis.

2. The ulcer history is of no relevance, but hypertrophic cardiomyopathy is an autosomal dominant trait with a high degree of penetrance. The sudden and unexplained death of the patient's father aged 48 could well have been caused by cardiomyopathy.

3. The gradient across the obstruction, and therefore the patient's murmur and symptoms, is increased by the Valsalva manoeuvre, by standing and by exercise. In contrast the gradient is decreased by the Mueller manoeuvre, and squatting.

4. ECG will show left ventricular hypertrophy and strain. Chest X-ray will show cardiomegaly with left ventricular prominence. Echocardiography is most useful in showing left ventricular hypertrophy of both posterior free wall and septum, left ventricular outflow obstruction and systolic anterior motion of the mitral valve as well as many other less common abnormalities.

5. FALSE   TRUE   FALSE   FALSE   FALSE

Acute rheumatic fever is rarely seen now in Western countries, and where it does occur it is usually in a modified, and milder, form. Nevertheless it is still a common illness in developing countries. The major Duckett-Jones criteria are carditis, arthritis, Sydenham's chorea, subcutaneous nodules and erythema marginatum.

6. TRUE   TRUE   TRUE   FALSE   FALSE

Where the heart is spared in the acute episode subsequent valvular heart disease is almost unknown. Where cardiac complications occur early they are usually due to severe mitral valve disease. Antistreptococcal antibiotics taken regularly in susceptible individuals prevent recurrence of acute rheumatic fever, the chances of developing a recurrence being increased by a previous attack. Restenosis of a mitral valve after valvotomy indicates continued scarring of a previously damaged valve rather than a fresh attack of rheumatic fever.

7. TRUE   TRUE   TRUE   FALSE   FALSE

The diagnosis of alcoholic cardiomyopathy may be difficult since stigmata of alcohol excess in other systems may be lacking and the patient may deny excess consumption. Abstention however may result in a return to complete cardiac normality. The illness may be punctuated by paroxysmal arrhythmia, including atrial fibrillation, and sudden death, and by systemic and pulmonary thromboembolism. Propranolol is contraindicated.

8. TRUE   FALSE   FALSE   TRUE   TRUE

The aetiology of cardiac myxoma is ill understood, some workers believing that it is the result of organized thrombus. It occurs most often in the atria, but 10% occur in ventricles. The lesion may be biatrial or biventricular. A familial association may exist. The commonest presentation is with features of mitral valve disease, but embolic phenomena are not uncommon. Rarely the patient may present with nonspecific compliants of pyrexia, weight loss, arthralgia, and rash, and may become cachectic.

9. TRUE FALSE TRUE TRUE TRUE

Aortic regurgitation, congenital or acquired (often as a consequence of infective endocarditis) is a not uncommon accompaniment of ventricular septal defect. Endocarditis is extremely rare following spontaneous closure of a ventricular septal defect, whereas it occurs in 4% of patients with a persistent abnormality especially in their third or fourth decades and often in the right ventricle opposite the 'jet' of blood coming through the defect. In tetralogy of Fallot, survival to adulthood in unoperated patients is possible because of the development of rich collaterals; temporary relief of dyspnoea is effected in children by squatting or less efficiently but with greater social acceptability by crossing the legs in adults. Biventricular hypertrophy is usually accompanied by large voltage complexes in right and left chest leads.

PATIENT 22

Answers are on pages 123–126

HISTORY

A 61 year old widow of Chilean extraction who has lived in this country for 15 years is admitted for elective cholecystectomy. However, since she is found to be in atrial fibrillation, a medical opinion is sought prior to surgery. On closer enquiry the patient admits to exertional dyspnoea for 10 years, and to prevent nocturnal dyspnoea sleeps with four pillows. She experiences chest discomfort radiating to the left arm on exertion but this usually responds to glyceryl trinitrate. For 20 years she has suffered from diabetes mellitus requiring oral hypoglycaemic drugs (currently chlorpropamide 250 mg daily and metformin 1 g daily). She smokes 15 cigarettes daily but is teetotal.

EXAMINATION

The patient speaks very poor English. Sallow complexion but no icterus. Marked bilateral pitting ankle oedema. JVP + 10 cm. Liver palpable 4 cm below right costal margin — non tender. No splenomegaly. No ascites. BP 190/110 mmHg in the right arm lying. Pulse — atrial fibrillation with a ventricular rate of 110/minute and a pulse deficit of 30/minute. Diffuse thrusting apical impulse in the fifth and sixth intercostal space in the anterior axillary line. Crowing 3/6 ejection systolic murmur at the base conducted to neck. Bilateral basal crepitations. Optic fundi — bilateral arteriovenous nipping, numerous haemorrhages and soft exudates between 4 and 8 o'clock in the right fundus. Neurological examination, as far as the patient is able to cooperate, is normal.

QUESTIONS

1. Which causes of heart disease are of possible relevance in this patient?

2. Indicate how each cause may contribute to cardiac problems.

3. How would you assess the relative contribution of each cause in this patient?

Multiple choice questions

4. Which of the following statements is/are true?

(a) *In a patient with atrial fibrillation whose ventricular rate is controlled at 60-80/minute with digoxin exercise will not alter the ventricular response.*

(b) *In atrial fibrillation the ventricular rate may be entirely regular.*

(c) *Failure to control the ventricular rate in a patient with congestive cardiac failure and atrial fibrillation by prescribing digoxin 0.25 mg bd. suggests that the dose usually requires to be increased.*

(c) *Verapamil orally may be used as the sole treatment to control the ventricular rate in a patient with atrial fibrillation who cannot tolerate digoxin.*

(e) *Atrial fibrillation may follow carotid sinus pressure in a patient with atrial flutter.*

5. In the Wolff-Parkinson-White syndrome:

(a) *Ebstein's anomaly of the tricuspid valve may be an associated feature*

(b) the reciprocating tachycardia usually passes antegradely along the accessory bundle and retrogradely through the A-V node
(c) amiodarone is the antiarrhythmic drug of choice
(d) digoxin may precipitate ventricular fibrillation in patients who have atrial fibrillation
(e) a negative delta wave in V1-V3, and a positive delta wave in V4-V6 implies an accessory pathway in the right ventricle.

6. A prolonged QT interval:

(a) may be associated with hereditary deafness
(b) may be produced by hypomagnesaemia
(c) signifies lignocaine toxicity
(d) is often associated with a prominent U wave
(e) may be a premorbid finding in young athletes who die suddenly.

7. Verapamil:

(a) has high first pass liver metabolism
(b) is contraindicated in bronchospasm
(c) was initially used as an alternative antianginal agent but is now thought to be of little value in this respect
(d) is useful in the management of patients with the sick sinus syndrome
(e) may be cautiously combined with digoxin in atrial fibrillation.

8. Which of the following statements regarding calcium antagonists is/are correct?

(a) Perhexilene, like nifedipine, is useful in the treatment of variant angina.
(b) Sublingual nifedipine may cause hypotension and collapse within 5 minutes of administration.

(c) *The dose of prenylamine may have to be moderated in patients receiving beta-blockers.*

(d) *Papilloedema is a recognized side effect of perhexilene.*

(e) *Verapamil in high dosage is effective in the symptomatic treatment of hypertrophic cardiomyopathy.*

ANSWERS AND DISCUSSIONS

PATIENT 22

1. Ischaemic heart disease
   Hypertensive heart disease
   Diabetes mellitus
   Trypanosomiasis (Chagas' disease).

2. Ischaemic heart disease may have caused her problems by precipitating biventricular failure, and through myocardial infarction with apical aneurysm formation.

   Hypertension would have contributed to ischaemic heart disease by accelerating atheroma deposition, and may have produced problems in its own right, namely left ventricular enlargement, and atrial fibrillation with consequent heart failure.

   Diabetes mellitus also accelerates atheroma deposition, but in that there is evidence in this patient of fundal microangiopathy diabetic cardiomyopathy is a possible contributory factor.

   Chagas' disease is a major cause of death in Chile and the chronic form of the trypanosomiasis appears a mean of 20 years after the initial infestation. Characteristic features are cardiomegaly, apical aneurysm, congestive heart failure and arrhythmias.

3. The relative contribution of hypertension may be roughly assessed by the presence of end organ damage — renal impairment (U & E), left ventricular hypertrophy (ECG) and hypertensive optic fundal changes. The relative contribution of diabetes is difficult to assess, but retinal microangiopathy is usually accompanied by microangiopathy elsewhere. Echocardiography may reveal features of congestive cardiomyopathy with apical aneurysm of Chagas' disease, while serology (Machado-Guerreiro complement — fixation text) may be helpful. However in a hypertensive diabetic smoker with apical dyskinesia, an ECG may reveal evidence of infarction with persistent ST elevation characteristic of ischaemic heart disease.

4. FALSE   TRUE   FALSE   TRUE   TRUE

Despite digitalization the A-V node is still under native sympathetic and vagal influences, and the ventricular response will therefore rise with exercise or emotion. Particularly with digoxin toxicity a nodal rhythm or complete heart block with a regular idioventricular rhythm and atrial fibrillation may coexist. Failure to control the ventricular rate with high doses of digoxin usually implies poor compliance, or nonabsorption of the drug from oedematous intestinal mucosa. Because it delays conduction at the A-V node verapamil may be used successfully to control the ventricular rate in atrial fibrillation. Carotid sinus pressure may convert atrial flutter to atrial fibrillation, or to sinus rhythm, may increase the degree of block while remaining in flutter, or have no effect.

5. TRUE   FALSE   TRUE   TRUE   TRUE

Anomalies associated with the W-P-W syndrome include Ebstein's anomaly of the tricuspid valve, mitral valve prolapse and cardiomyopathy. Though while the patient is in sinus rhythm the atrial impulses pass antegradely via the accessory bundle to the ventricles in supraventricular tachycardia the conduction is usually antegrade by the A-V node and retrograde via the accessory bundle — thus patients presenting with supraventricular tachycardia secondary to W-P-W syndrome may not be recognized as such until they revert to sinus rhythm. Amiodarone is probably the most helpful antiarrhythmic agent in W-P-W syndrome. Digoxin may accelerate antegrade conduction in atrial fibrillation and the more rapid the ventricular response the greater the danger of developing ventricular tachycardia or fibrillation. Type B W-P-W with delta waves negative in V1-V3 and positive in V4-V6 implies a right ventricular accessory pathway.

6. TRUE   TRUE   FALSE   TRUE   TRUE

A prolonged QT interval is associated with an increased risk of collapse or sudden death due to ventricular tachydysrrhythmias and may be a cause of unexpected death in young athletes. A prolonged interval may be found as a hereditary disorder accompanying congenital deafness but is more commonly the result of electrolyte disorders (such as hypokalaemia or hypomagnesaemia), drugs (such as quinidine, not lignocaine, or phenothiazines) or neurological upset (stroke or head trauma). A prominent U wave also accompanies hypokalaemia.

7. TRUE   FALSE   FALSE   FALSE   TRUE

First pass liver metabolism is high with verapamil, hence the differential between the intravenous and oral doses. The drug may be used safely in patients with bronchospasm. Verapamil is still used to good effect in angina pectoris though other calcium antagonists, particularly nifedipine, are of greater potency in this respect. Since verapamil increases block at the A-V node it is potentially hazardous in the sick sinus syndrome. Since verapamil and digoxin may have toxic effects on the conducting system great care must be exercised where they are used in combination.

8. FALSE   TRUE   TRUE   TRUE   TRUE

Perhexilene differs from verapamil and nifedipine in being ineffective in Prinzmetal angina; though it is effective in stable angina it has troublesome side effects including ataxia, liver disease, peripheral neuropathy and rarely papilloedema. Prenylamine is an antianginal agent with some calcium antagonist properties, which also causes peripheral vasodilation, hypotension and myocardial depression, such that the dosage must be moderated if beta-blockers are added. Verapamil has been claimed to be the most effective symptomatic treatment in hypertrophic cardiomyopathy. It is useful to assess those patients who are going to have a marked hypotensive response to nifedipine by observing the rapid effects of a sublingual dose of the drug.

PATIENT 23

Answers are on pages 130–132

HISTORY

A 58 year old crofter presents with a fractured ulna after slipping on some ice. His general practitioner finding his blood pressure to be consistently raised refers him for further assessment. The patient, who has no past medical history of note, complaints of occasional occipital headache, episodic epigastric discomfort related to the ingestion of fatty foods, and some dysuria without frequency, hesitancy or haematuria.

EXAMINATION

On examination his BP is 230/130 mmHg, and he has atrial fibrillation with a ventricular rate of 80 beats/minute. Arteriovenous nipping is the only abnormality detected on optic fundal examination. The cardiac apex is in the 6th intercostal space in the anterior axillary line. There is no left ventricular failure.

INITIAL INVESTIGATIONS

Serum electrolytes — sodium 137 mmol/1, potassium 3.8 mmol/1, bicarbonate 26 mmol/1. Haemoglobin 12.3 g/dl.

ESR 44 mm in one hour. Electrocardiogram shows left ventricular hypertrophy and strain. Intravenous urography — right kidney measures 13.6 cm in bipolar diameter and the left 7.0 cm. Contrast is very poorly excreted by the left kidney.

QUESTIONS

1. What further investigations, if any, are indicated?

2. What is the differential diagnosis?

3. The patient's blood pressure is not satisfactorily controlled by beta-blocker, diuretic and prazosin, and the question of left nephrectomy has been raised; what is your opinion of this?

4. Are there any precautions you would take at the time of surgery?

Multiple choice questions

5. The following are helpful symptoms in a hypertensive patient with respect to the aetiology of the hypertension:

(a) *dizziness*

(b) *loin pain of sudden onset*

(c) *nocturnal diarrhoea*

(d) *obstipation*

(e) *muscle cramps*

6. In the radiological investigation of the renal status of a hypertensive patient:

(a) *the size of an individual kidney may be observed to change by as much as 2.0 cm during the course of an intravenous urogram*

(b) *cortical scarring always signifies previous infection of the renal parenchyma*

(c) *absence of contrast from the expected site of one kidney 10 minutes after injection of contrast in an i.v.u. is persuasive evidence that the kidney is absent*

(d) *erect and supine abdominal films may demonstrate nephroptosis only in parous women.*

(d) *arteriography may precipitate acute renal failure.*

7. Unilateral nephrectomy restores normal blood pressure in the great majority of patients with the following conditions?:

(a) *hydronephrosis*

(b) *pyelonephritis*

(c) *renal artery occlusion*

(d) *renal tuberculosis*

(e) *renal artery stenosis.*

8. Which of the following statements is/are true of prazosin?

(a) *Its primary mode of action is as a peripheral vasodilator.*

(b) *Unexpected hypotensive episodes are rare but may occur at any time during treatment.*

(c) *It may have a synergistic effect when used in combination with hydrallazine.*

(d) *It may precipitate urinary retention.*

(e) *Tachyphylaxis is extremely rare.*

9. The finding of a small (less than 9.0 cm in bipolar diameter) kidney implies:

(a) *that the kidney is functionally abnormal*

(b) *that creatinine clearance in that kidney will be reduced*

(c) *that the contralateral kidney is likely to be enlarged (greater than 14 cm)*

(d) *that plasma renin concentration in the renal vein blood will be increased*

(e) *that urine flow rate will be reduced compared with a contralateral kidney which is 12 cm in bipolar diameter.*

ANSWERS AND DISCUSSION

PATIENT 23

1. Mid-stream specimen of urine for culture and sensitivity. Early morning specimens of urine for culture for alcohol and acid fast bacilli. Sputum culture for alcohol and acid fast bacilli. Mantoux test. Chest X-ray. Creatinine clearance. Plasma renin angiotensin II and aldosterone concentrations. Renal arteriography. Renal vein sampling.

2. Renal artery stenosis or occlusion
Renal artery embolism in view of the cardiac rhythm, but there is no history to support an embolic event
Renal tuberculosis
Ask-Upmark kidney
Small kidney of undetermined aetiology

3. There is nothing to be lost by left nephrectomy if the left kidney is not contributing to renal function. However the overall renal impairment and cardiomegaly with left ventricular hypertrophy all point to hypertension of longstanding. These findings are against surgery returning blood pressure to normal. It may, however, make antihypertensive control easier.

It should be noted that a full trial of medical management has not been made. Both minoxidil and captopril in combination with diuretics and in the case of minoxidil betablockers would probably control this patient's blood pressure.

If the diagnosis is tuberculosis surgery is indicated.

4. If tuberculosis has not been excluded antituberculous drugs should precede surgery and be continued until histology is available. If plasma angiotensin II concentrations are high and the plasma renin concentration in renal vein blood from the small kidney is very high then a precipitate fall in blood pressure at nephrectomy may occur. Agents to maintain blood pressure such as angiotensin should ideally be available

5. FALSE   TRUE   FALSE   TRUE   TRUE

Loin pain of sudden onset may indicate the presence of renal infarction, renal stones, or rupture of a cyst in a patient with polycystic kidneys. Obstipation may be a notable complaint in patients with phaeochromocytoma but this may partly be related to the drugs required to treat the condition. Muscle cramps are a common finding in hyperaldosteronism and may be a helpful if nonspecific pointer to the diagnosis. Dizziness and nocturnal diarrhoea do not help in determining the cause of a patient's hypertension.

6. TRUE   FALSE   FALSE   FALSE   TRUE

The size of a kidney may change by as much as 2.0 cm during the osmotic load at intravenous urography, particularly where an oral water load is given in addition. Cortical scarring may signify previous infarction as well as infection. In severe renal artery stenosis or renal artery occlusion contrast may appear even later than 10 minutes after the injection of contrast but even if it does not appear at all this does not imply that the kidney is absent altogether. Nephroptosis is not an uncommon finding particularly in tall people of both sexes and all degrees of parity; its relevance to renal disease is disputed.

Arteriography may precipitate renal failure either through a severe allergic response, or by causing spasm or thrombus formation over a renal artery stenosis, the contralateral renal artery being occluded.

7. FALSE   FALSE   FALSE   FALSE   FALSE

In no surgically correctable cause of hypertension is normal blood pressure restored in the great majority of patients. Most experience has been gained with renal artery stenosis and adrenal adenomata and in both of these conditions normal blood pressure is restored in approximately half of the surgically treated patients. A further third is improved, i.e., less in the way of antihypertensive therapy is required to control blood pressure postoperatively. The remainder are not improved by surgery.

8. FALSE TRUE TRUE FALSE FALSE

The primary mode of action of prazosin is as a postsynaptic alpha-receptor blocker. It may produce unexpected hypotensive episodes at any time during the course of treatment though particularly with the first dose but this is not a common side effect. Since its mode of action is different from the arteriolar vasodilatation of hydrallazine a synergistic effect may be found. Prazosin has not been found to be associated with urinary retention. Tachyphylaxis is not uncommon but responsiveness of the patient may be regained by the addition of a more potent diuretic to the regimen.

9. FALSE TRUE TRUE FALSE TRUE

A small kidney is not necessarily functionally abnormal. Its overall contribution to creatinine clearance even with normal function is less than that of the contralateral kidney, which is likely to have undergone compensatory hypertrophy if the abnormality has been present since birth. Urine flow rate will be reduced in the small kidney and in the absence of other pathology plasma renin concentration in renal vein blood will be normal.

PATIENT 24

Answers are on pages 135–137

HISTORY

A 48 year old housewife has been attending the cardiology outpatient clinic at 2 yearly intervals since discovery of a murmur during the last of three pregnancies at age 35. Over the 19 months since her last review she has experienced many episodes of palpitation and dyspnoea. For 12 months dyspnoea has been marked on climbing one flight of stairs and she has had to seek the aid of her relations to get her housework and shopping done. She has required to sleep with three pillows, and she has been troubled by an irritating unproductive cough especially at night. She has not experienced chest pain or episodes of altered consciousness. For three months, however, she has been continuously hoarse, and has given up smoking 20 cigarettes daily as a consequence. She has been referred back to the cardiology clinic following ENT opinion which has demonstrated paralysis of the left vocal cord.

QUESTIONS

1. What explanations can you offer for this sequence of events?

2. Which two initial investigations will you find most helpful?

Multiple choice questions

3. Survival into adulthood is expected in patients with:

(a) ventricular septal defect with pulmonary stenosis

(b) tricuspid atresia

(c) persistent ductus arteriosus

(d) ventricular septal defect with aortic regurgitaion

(e) ostium secundum atrial septal defect.

4. Which of the following statements is/are true?

(a) Patients with congenital pulmonary stenosis may develop angina pectoris with normal coronary arteries.

(b) Congenital stenosis of peripheral pulmonary arteries is not unexpected after the rubella syndrome in pregnancy.

(c) Prominent pulmonary arteries may be associated with pulmonary stenosis.

(d) Differential cyanosis and infective endocarditis of the pulmonary artery may coexist in patients with persistent ductus arteriosus.

(e) Rheumatic mitral stenosis and congenital atrial septal defect constitute a well recognized syndrome.

5. Patients with atrial septal defect:

(a) may present for the first time at age 50 with congestive cardiac failure

(b) usually develop pulmonary hypertension more quickly if they live at high altitude

(c) who have an early diastolic murmur probably have regurgitation of a coexistent congenitally abnormal aortic valve

(d) with electrocardiographic evidence of right bundle branch block and left axis deviation usually have secundum defects

(e) should have the defect closed even in the fifth decade if the pulmonary to systemic flow exceeds a ratio of 2:1.

6. Paradoxical embolism may occur in patients with:

(a) *persistent ductus arteriosus*

(b) *atrial septal defect*

(c) *patent foramen ovale*

(d) *Ebstein's anomaly*

(e) *ventricular septal defect.*

7. A mid-diastolic murmur may occur in:

(a) *tricuspid regurgitation*

(b) *right atrial tumour*

(c) *thyrotoxicosis*

(d) *acute rheumatic fever*

(e) *left atrial tumour*

ANSWERS AND DISCUSSION

PATIENT 24

1. The initial discovery of a murmur during pregnancy, the long follow up without surgical intervention and the progressive dyspnoea all suggest deteriorating mitral stenosis. Where the left atrium is greatly enlarged it may produce a recurrent laryngeal nerve palsy by pushing up the left pulmonary artery which compresses the nerve against the arch of the aorta. Alternative explanations are an expanding aortic aneurysm causing the palsy, or bronchial carcinoma in a smoker affecting the recurrent laryngeal nerve, but these alternatives ignore the slowly progressive nature of this patient's illness.

2. Most helpful initially would be chest X–ray and echocardiography.

3. TRUE FALSE TRUE FALSE TRUE

Patients with ventricular septal defect with pulmonary stenosis, with persistent ductus arteriosus, and with ostium secundum atrial septal defects often survive to adulthood, but are liable to endocarditis and to development of the Eisenmenger syndrome as time advances. An atretic tricuspid valve, and the combination of a ventricular septal defect with aortic regurgitation usually results in early demise.

4. TRUE TRUE TRUE FALSE TRUE

In pulmonary stenosis angina may result from undue demands on the arterial supply by a hypertrophied right ventricle. After rubella a number of cardiac anomalies may occur — persistent ductus arteriosus, atrial and ventricular septal defects, Fallot's tetralogy, supravalvar aortic stenosis, and stenosis of the peripheral pulmonary arteries. Post-stenotic dilatation of the main pulmonary artery and left pulmonary artery is often visible on the chest X–ray of patients with pulmonary stenosis. Differential cyanosis in persistent ductus arteriosus implies shunting of venous blood to the lower half of the body while endocarditis of the pulmonary artery usually implies reversed shunting: the two are therefore very unlikely to occur simultaneously. Lutembacher's syndrome consists of congenital atrial septal defect and rheumatic mitral stenosis but why these occur together is not clearly understood.

5. TRUE TRUE FALSE FALSE TRUE

Patients with atrial septal defect may remain asymptomatic for decades before presenting with cardiac failure. Patients who live at sea level rarely develop pulmonary hypertension before the age of 20, whereas this is not uncommon in those living at high altitudes. An early diastolic murmur is more likely to arise from the pulmonary valve in patients with pulmonary hypertension. Right bundle branch block is characteristic in atrial septal defect, with right axis deviation in secundum defects and left axis deviation in primum defects. If pulmonary hypertension has not yet developed and the shunt is significant even elderly patients benefit from surgery.

6. TRUE   TRUE   TRUE   FALSE   TRUE

Paradoxical embolism may occur where a cardiac defect allows the pulmonary circulation to be bypassed, i.e. patent foramen orale, atrial septal defect, ventricular septal defect, and persistent ductus arteriosus. Reversal of the direction of the shunt usually occurs first. In Ebstein's anomaly no shunt exists.

7. FALSE   TRUE   TRUE   TRUE   TRUE

Tricuspid regurgitation produces a systolic murmur. Atrial myxoma, be it left or right sided, mimics mitral stenosis with diastolic murmurs often present. In high output states such as thyrotoxicosis increased flow across a normal mitral valve may produce a diastolic murmur. In acute rheumatic fever with valvulitis the so-called Carey-Coombs' murmur may occur.

PATIENT 25

Answers are on pages 141–143

HISTORY

A 70 year old retired miner is referred to the medical outpatient clinic for investigation of exertional dyspnoea, cough and ½ stone weight loss over a 6 months period. He does not experience chest pain. In the past he has suffered from pulmonary tuberculosis (age 26), underwent left inguinal herniorrhaphy (age 54) and underwent resection of the descending colon (age 60) because of obstruction secondary to extensive diverticular disease. Despite his presenting complaints he smokes 5 cigarettes daily though formerly 30/day. He takes slow release aminophylline 2 tablets twice daily, prednisolone 5 mg daily, and uses a salbutamol inhaler 2 puffs four times daily.

EXAMINATION

He is short (5′ 2″) and thin (50 kg) with audible wheeze. Poor chest expansion: widespread rhonchi. BP 160/90 mmHg in the right arm, lying. Pulse — atrial fibrillation, ventricular rate 100/min. Heart sounds pure. No murmurs. Abdominal examination normal. He is mentally confused especially with regard to time and place.
    He has no close relatives and lives alone. You decide to admit him for further investigation.

INITIAL INVESTIGATIONS

Hb 12.6 g/dl, WBC 6.9 × 10^9/l, ESR = 40 mm in one hour. Urea 8.3 mmol/l, Na 134 mmol/l, K 3.5 mmol/l. Thyroxine 130 nmol/l. ALT 46 U/l. AST 35 U/l. LDH 305 U/l. Total protein 66 g/l. Albumin 31 g/l. ECG — atrial fibrillation, T inversion in I, aVL, V5, V6. Chest X-ray — emphysema with fibrotic changes at the left apex.

QUESTIONS

1. What explanations can you offer for the patient's weight loss?

2. What explanations can you offer for the arrhythmia?

3. Why is the patient confused?

Multiple choice questions

4. A low voltage ECG may occur in patients with:

(a) *hypopituitarism*

(b) *achondroplasia*

(c) *obesity*

(d) *emphysema*

(e) *digoxin toxicity.*

5. A technetium pyrophosphate scan:

(a) *is invariably normal after cardioversion unless a patient has suffered a myocardial infarction*

(b) *may be positive in patients with calcific mitral stenosis*

(c) *is more sensitive than an exercise tolerance test in detecting significant coronary artery disease*

(d) *usually clears within 48 hours*

(e) *may be used to diagnose a right ventricular infarction.*

6. Potential hazards of coronary angiography include:

(a) *hypovolaemic shock*

(b) *anaphylactic shock*

(c) *ventricular fibrillation*

(d) *myocardial infarction*

(e) *disseminated intravascular coagulation.*

7. Paradoxical splitting of the second heart sound is found in:

(a) *temporary right ventricular pacing*

(b) *pulmonary embolism*

(c) *ventricular septal defect*

(d) *left bundle branch block*

(e) *Wolff-Parkinson-White syndrome Type A.*

8. Permanent ventricular demand (VVI) pacemakers:

(a) *may be inhibited by microwave ovens*

(b) *form an absolute contraindication to diathermy*

(c) *when accompanied by twitching of the patient's left shoulder should be replaced*

(d) *may become faulty because patients 'twiddle' with the electrode*

(e) *may precipitate cardiac failure.*

ANSWERS AND DISCUSSION

PATIENT 25

1. Many possible explanations could be put forward for this man's weight loss. Active consideration should be given to:
   - (a) the weight loss that accompanies chronic obstructive airways disease
   - (b) thyrotoxicosis (a TRH test may yield a flat TSH response even where serum thyroxine is within recognized 'normal' limits)
   - (c) reactivation of pulmonary tuberculosis by steroids
   - (d) bronchial carcinoma (smoking habits)
   - (e) secondary bowel carcinoma (the original operation may have been for colonic neoplasm despite what the patient was told)
   - (f) malnourishment in a chronic abuser of alcohol
   - (g) prolonged theophylline toxicity with nausea and vomiting.

2. Atrial fibrillation may be the result of:
   - (a) ischaemic heart disease
   - (b) degenerative heart disease
   - (c) thyrotoxicosis
   - (d) theophylline toxicity
   - (e) tumour infiltrating the heart.

3. Confusion may be due to:
   - (a) cerebral hypoxia
   - (b) alcohol withdrawal
   - (c) arteriosclerotic dementia
   - (d) thyrotoxicosis
   - (e) theophylline toxicity.

4. TRUE   FALSE   TRUE   TRUE   FALSE

Low voltage ECGs may occur in emphysema, obesity, pericardial effusion, constrictive pericarditis, myxoedema and rarely in hypopituitarism. Voltage may appear to be low if there is incorrect standardization, and in achondroplasia the patient is low, not his ECG voltage.

5. FALSE   TRUE   FALSE   FALSE   TRUE

Infarct-avid scans performed using Tc pyrophosphate may be falsely positive after repeated high-voltage cardioversion, and since the radiopharmaceutical is also bone-avid in calcific mitral stenosis also. Scintigraphy is not the investigation of choice in diagnosing myocardial ischaemia, but is useful in detecting infarction of both left and right ventricles. In the majority of patients who have suffered an acute myocardial infarction the scan is still abnormal 1 or 2 weeks later.

6. TRUE   TRUE   TRUE   TRUE   FALSE

Though coronary angiography is potentially hazardous, in many respects problems rarely occur. If excessive unrecognized bleeding occurs at the femoral artery puncture site, symptoms and signs of acute blood loss may develop. Allergic reactions to contrast are usually minor but potentially fatal. Equipment for cardioversion should be readily available at all catheter laboratories. Dislodgement of thrombus or the prolonged presence of a catheter in a compromised coronary artery may precipitate infarction.

7. TRUE   FALSE   FALSE   TRUE   FALSE

Paradoxical splitting of the second heart sound (i.e. P_2 before A_2) may be caused by delay in A_2 or an early P_2. Delay in A_2 may be the result of delayed activation and contraction of the left ventricle as in left bundle branch block or a right ventricular pacemaker, or the result of prolonged systole as in myocardial infarction or aortic regurgitation. An early P_2 occurs in W-P-W syndrome type B, where there is early activation of the right ventricle.

8. TRUE FALSE FALSE TRUE TRUE

VVI pacemakers (Ventricle paced, Ventricle sensed, mode of response Inhibition) may be temporarily inhibited while the patient is in close proximity to equipment producing high frequency waves, such as microwave ovens. Diathermy if performed close to a pacemaker may result in the current being channelled through the electrode; diathermy of the prostate gland seems to be relatively safe. Twitching of the patient's shoulder usually demands better insulation of the pulse generator, not its replacement. Among the many causes of pacemaker malfunction is fracture of the electrode at the shoulder following prolonged twiddling by the patient. If ventricular pacing occurs in a patient with borderline cardiac function such that the atrial 'kick' which may contribute 30% or 40% to cardiac output in these circumstances is lost then cardiac failure may be precipitated — the 'pacemaker syndrome'.

PATIENT 26

Answers are on pages 147–149

HISTORY

A 45 year old labourer who is known to have been hypertensive for 2 years presents with a 2 month history of frontal headache, deteriorating vision, and transient episodes of weakness, palpitation, tremor, pallor, nausea and vomiting. He is a 20/day cigarette smoker and drinks 6 pints of lager each night. Drugs on admission — methyldopa 750 mg daily. He gives no other past history of note.

EXAMINATION

On examination the patient is plethoric and anxious. BP 240/146 mmHg. Optic fundal examination shows bilateral haemorrhages exudates and papilloedema. Pulse 60/min, regular. Abdominal examination normal. Gait is mildly ataxic with slight hyperreflexia in the legs and Chaddock's sign is positive bilaterally though both plantar responses are flexor.

INITIAL INVESTIGATIONS

Haemoglobin 12.8 g/dl. Serum electrolytes: sodium 138 mmol/l, potassium 3.7 mmol/l, bicarbonate 28 mmol/l; urea 6.6 mmol/l, creatinine 102 μmol/l. Creatinine clearance 96 ml/min.

QUESTIONS

1. What is the differential diagnosis?

2. What explanations can you offer for the neurological signs?

3. What investigations do you think will clarify the picture?

4. What would be your initial and longterm management?

Multiple choice questions

5. In diagnosing phaeochromocytoma:

(a) *urinary normetadrenaline estimations are rarely influenced by drug treatment*

(b) *glucose intolerance is a common associated finding*

(c) *vena caval sampling is a helpful manoeuvre*

(d) *arteriography often precipitates a hypertensive crisis*

(e) *the presence of normal plasma concentrations of noradrenaline and adrenaline and of urinary concentrations of catecholamine breakdown products satisfactorily excludes the diagnosis.*

6. Cerebral haemorrhage is a common morbid event in hypertension; which of the following statements concerning cerebral haemorrhage is/are true?

(a) *its incidence may be reduced by successful blood pressure control*

(b) *the risk of stroke is related to systolic blood pressure even at levels below 140 mmHg*

(c) *ruptured berry aneurysm is a recognized complication in polycystic kidney disease*

(d) *it may not be possible to distinguish cerebral haemorrhage from hypertensive encephalopathy*

(e) *all patients with a diastolic pressure of greater than 120 mmHg. at presentation with a stroke should be treated with hypotensive drugs within 12 hours of admission*

7. Sustained blood pressure elevation may have the following effects on the eye:

(a) uveitis

(b) haemorrhages and exudates in the retina due to leakage of blood and plasma

(c) optic atrophy

(d) cataract

(e) bilateral papilloedema without haemorrhages or exudates

8. The following are common side effects of the named oral hypotensive agents?

(a) nightmares — atenolol

(b) diarrhoea — guanethidine

(c) postural dizziness — bethanidine

(d) hirsutism — diazoxide

(e) nasal congestion — reserpine

9. The following are recognized associations of phaeochromocytoma:

(a) anaemia

(b) medullary carcinoma of the thyroid

(c) postural hypotension

(d) normotension

(e) myocarditis.

GREY CASES 147

ANSWERS AND DISCUSSION

PATIENT 26

1. Malignant phase hypertension secondary either to phaeochromocytoma or to essential hypertension; intracranial space occupying lesion.

2. Either small brain stem infarcts (etat lacunaire) secondary to malignant phase hypertension or a space occupying lesion in the region of the fourth ventricle.

3. Urinary normetadrenaline concentration
   Plasma adrenaline and noradrenaline levels during an attack .
   Computerized tomography of the abdomen looking for a lesion of the adrenal or extraadrenal chromaffin tissue
   Skull X-rays
   Electroencephalogram
   Computerized tomography of head — ?posterior fossa lesion

4. Labetalol or phenoxybenzamine/beta-blocker combination.
Note: This patient suffered from a syndrome known as a pseudophaeochromocytoma where symptoms of a phaeochromocytoma are mimicked by a posterior fossa lesion. The differential diagnosis is complicated by the existence of the Von Hippel-Lindau syndrome (cerebelloretinal haemangioblastomatosis) which may be accompanied by a phaeochromocytoma. In this patient's case there was histological evidence of the changes of malignant phase hypertension in his kidneys at postmortem, but he also had a cerebellar haemangioblastoma without retinal haemangiomata or phaeochromocytoma.

5. FALSE   TRUE   TRUE   TRUE   FALSE

Unfortunately many antihypertensive drugs influence urinary normetadrenaline levels. Plasma adrenaline and noradrenaline levels are more direct tests but even they may be normal between phaeochromocytoma attacks; samples obtained during an attack will be diagnostic. Vena caval sampling may be a helpful diagnostic procedure in localizing the lesion, but it has largely been superceded by computerized tomography. Arteriography may be an unhappily dramatic diagnostic test, often undertaken unwittingly in a patient with suspected renovascular hypertension. Phaeochromocytoma patients are often thin individuals with glucose intolerance, a reflection of their hypercatabolic state.

6. TRUE   TRUE   TRUE   TRUE   FALSE

The incidence of stroke is reduced by successful blood pressure control; surprisingly the evidence in favour of a similar reduction in the incidence of myocardial infarction is tenuous. The risk of stroke is related to systolic pressure even at levels within the accepted normal range. Ruptured berry aneurysms are more common in both polycystic kidney disease and coarctation of the aorta. Hypertensive encephalopathic changes with swelling of the brain tissue may be one cause of stroke, though with control of blood pressure the neurological signs may resolve. Hypertension in the early hours and days after a stroke is not uncommon and often settles spontaneously; unless other evidence of premorbid hypertension is available early treatment is not indicated.

7. FALSE   TRUE   FALSE   FALSE   TRUE

Uveitis, optic atrophy and cataract are not direct consequences of sustained blood pressure elevation. Haemorrhages and exudates in the retina are caused by leakage of blood and plasma and signify malignant phase hypertension. Bilateral papilloedema is also indicative of malignant phase hypertension and may occur in the absence of haemorrhages or exudates.

8. FALSE TRUE TRUE TRUE TRUE

Atenolol is relatively free from the cerebral side effects such as nightmares of the less hydrophilic betablockers such as propranolol. Diarrhoea and failure of ejaculation are common problems with guanethidine related to its effect on the autonomic nervous system. Likewise bethanidine, a related adrenergic neurone blocker, commonly causes postural hypotension. Hirsutism is a common side effect with oral diazoxide as it is with minoxidil. Nasal congestion is among the many side effects of the Rauwolfia alkaloid reserpine which acts by depleting the postganglionic adrenergic neurones of noradrenaline.

9. FALSE TRUE TRUE TRUE TRUE

Finding normal blood pressure between hypertensive attacks is not uncommon in patients with phaeochromocytoma. However, many patients have sustained hypertension in addition to episodic symptoms. 10% of adrenal medullary tumours (which themselves account for 90% of all phaeochromocytomas) are bilateral and multiple adrenal tumours are especially common in patients with simple familial phaeochromocytoma or one of the pluriglandular syndromes such as multiple endocrine adenomatosis Type II (Sipple's syndrome) which is associated with medullary carcinoma of the thyroid gland. Myocarditis is not an uncommon finding in patients dying with phaeochromocytoma, and the inflammatory changes are thought to be due to the high circulating catecholamine levels since a similar picture can be induced in experimental animals. Anaemia is not a well recognized finding.

PATIENT 27

Answers are on pages 153–155

HISTORY

A 54 year old fisherman has been flown to hospital by helicopter after the sudden onset at sea of left sided chest pain and sweating especially of the trunk, apparently precipitated by a fit of coughing. His general health has been poor for several months with vague chest discomfort often precipitated by vigorous exertion, and irritating unproductive cough for several years. He has been hypertensive for 10 years and claims to be taking clonidine and bendrofluazide. His only other complaint is of poor balance with a tendency, in the last 2 weeks, to stagger to the left. He smokes 30 cigarettes daily and drinks spirits, averaging 2 bottles per week.

EXAMINATION

On admission he is hypotensive (blood pressure 100/60) with sinus tachycardia (110/minute). Heart sounds normal. Coarse crepitations at both bases, right more than left. Liver edge palpable and slightly tender 3 cm below the right costal margin. Neurological examination — impaired heel-shin testing on the left; reflexes symmetrical; plantars flexor.

ECG shows symmetrical T wave inversion in the lateral chest leads.

QUESTIONS

1. The admitting resident thinks that the patient has suffered a subendocardial myocardial infarction. What other diagnoses, if any, would you consider?

2. Chest X–ray shows cardiomegaly, prominent vascular shadows, and interstitial pulmonary oedema. Do these findings allow you to exclude any of the diagnoses you have considered?

3. AST is 240 U/l and LDH 408 U/l — do these results substantiate the resident's diagnosis?

Multiple choice questions

4. Following blunt chest trauma:

(a) *atrial fibrillation usually reverts to sinus rhythm within 4 weeks*

(b) *myocardial infarction may occur in the absence of abnormal coronary arteries*

(c) *pericarditis nearly always occurs*

(d) *acute mitral regurgitation is the commonest valvular lesion*

(e) *arrhythmias are uncommon.*

5. In pericarditis:

(a) *the pain is largely due to associated pleurisy since the pericardium is itself largely insensitive to pain*

(b) *dyspnoea associated with relief of pain often signifies the development of a pericardial effusion*

(c) *the patient often experiences relief from pain by sitting up and leaning forward*

(d) *chest X-ray is of little diagnostic value.*

(e) *the ECG is always abnormal.*

6. Pericardiocentesis:

(a) *should be performed with the patient flat and sedated*

(b) *should ideally be performed with a needle attached to a chest lead of the ECG*

(c) *may be aided as a diagnostic test by gas analysis of aspirate*

(d) *is best performed with a number 16 French gauge needle*

(e) *is contraindicated in patients on warfarin therapy.*

7. Calf discomfort on exertion may occur in patients with:

(a) *erythromelalgia*

(b) *Buerger's disease*

(c) *persistent ductus arteriosus*

(d) *antihypertensive treatment (no beta-blockers)*

(e) *amyloidosis.*

8. Which of the following statements is/are true?

(a) *Venography of the calves is a thrombogenic procedure.*

(b) *Scanning of the legs after injection of ^{125}I-fibrinogen provides a rapid diagnostic test for deep venous thrombosis.*

(c) *Warfarin is the safest anticoagulant to use in the first trimester of pregnancy.*

(d) *Hypertensive patients are proven to be at higher risk from the haemorrhagic complications of anticoagulants than are normotensive patients.*

(e) *Elevated fibrin degradation products are a valuable aid to the diagnosis of deep venous thrombosis.*

ANSWERS AND DISCUSSION

PATIENT 27

1. The history of prolonged ill health, smoking and unproductive cough raises the possibilities of bronchial neoplasm, or with his alcohol history of pulmonary tuberculosis. The sudden onset of chest pain after coughing suggests pneumothorax, while the history of ataxia, proprioceptive loss and chest pain with trunk sweating after coughing suggest tumour in the thoracic spine with vertebral body collapse.

2. The chest X–ray appearances may be of longstanding in a patient with chronic ischaemic heart disease and/or hypertension. The absence of pneumothorax, evidence of tuberculosis, and neoplasm on the initial film make these diagnoses unlikely but have not absolutely excluded them.

3. One set of enzyme results does not allow conclusions to be reached about myocardial infarction, particularly since the patient drinks heavily and has hepatomegaly. The resident's diagnosis may prove to be correct, but the history is atypical. A further explanation of these enzymes is that they are the result of liver metastases in keeping with vertebral metastases — liver scan or ultrasound and thoracic spine X–rays and bone scan will be useful arbiters.

4. TRUE   TRUE   TRUE   FALSE   FALSE

As a result of blunt chest trauma myocardial contusion or infarction may occur in the absence of coronary artery disease, transient arrhythmias such as atrial fibrillation are common while more sinister early arrhythmias such as ventricular tachycardia may occur; mild acute pericarditis commonly occurs (rarely as a result of haemopericardium), and valvular damage may occur, most commonly of the aortic valve.

5. TRUE   TRUE   TRUE   TRUE   FALSE

Only a small area of the lower parietal pericardium (supplied by the phrenic nerve) is pain sensitive, and thus most pain in pericarditis is the result of associated pleurisy. When the inflamed pleural surfaces are separate by an effusion relief of pain usually occurs; and shifting pericardial fluid to the inflamed area by sitting up and leaning forward may relieve pain and ease dyspnoea. The chest X–ray is usually unhelpful in confirming the diagnosis and though the ECG is commonly abnormal it is still unhelpful in around one fifth of cases.

6. FALSE   TRUE   TRUE   FALSE   FALSE

Pericardial aspiration should be performed with the patient propped at 45°, and premedication is usually unnecessary. A fine gauge needle is used (19 or 21 gauge), and ECG monitoring from the needle tip is highly desirable and simple to perform. If a haemorrhagic effusion is aspirated it may not be immediately clear whether the aspirate is pure blood from a cardiac chamber or haemorrhagic effusion — the latter will not usually clot in a glass tube, and the pCO_2 will be higher and the pH lower than in arterial blood. Invasive procedures are clearly undesirable in anticoagulated patients, but warfarin therapy is certainly not an absolute contraindication to pericardiocentesis.

7. FALSE   TRUE   TRUE   TRUE   FALSE

Thromboangiitis obliterans (Buerger's disease) is an inflammatory disorder of the peripheral arteries and veins of male heavy smokers — the usual symptoms affect the feet or digits but may affect the calf. With reversed shunting in patients with persistent ductus arteriosus and pulmonary hypertension, desaturated blood flows principally to the legs (differential cyanosis) and patients complain of leg fatigue particularly on exertion. Any successful antihypertensive treatment may reduce blood flow through a critical stenosis such that distal ischaemia develops. In erythromelalgia burning or itching of the feet occurs as ambient temperature rises — the phenomenon is ill understood, but may respond to aspirin or indomethacin.

8. TRUE FALSE FALSE FALSE FALSE

Venography is an irritant thrombogenic procedure and patients should ideally be anticoagulated beforehand. Because ^{125}I-fibrinogen must be incorporated in thrombus before a positive scan can develop the procedure takes time, and does not provide a speedy test for deep venous thrombosis. Estimation of fibrinogen/fibrin degradation products has low specificity and sensitivity as a diagnostic test. Warfarin may be teratogenic especially in the first trimester of pregnancy such that if anticoagulation is necessary heparin should be used. There is no reliable evidence currently available that hypertensive patients on anticoagulants are more prone to haemorrhagic complications.

PATIENT 28

Answers are on pages 159–161

HISTORY

A 50 year old farm labourer presents to the accident and emergency department after 90 minutes of retrosternal tightness radiating to this throat which developed while he was baling hay. He has experienced many similar but shorter episodes of discomfort following vigorous exercise over the previous year but these have been relieved by rest. Eight years previously he underwent cardiac surgery but he is not very clear what this involved. He smokes 20 cigarettes daily but laughingly tells you that doctors have tried to stop him smoking many times without success. Furthermore he drinks as much spirits as he can afford, usually around 1½ bottles of whisky per week. His father suffered from diabetes mellitus while his mother died aged 76 after a 'heart attack'. The patient also confesses to nocturia (x2), and to discomfort in his right knee in the mornings.

EXAMINATION

He is a stocky plethoric individual. Peripheral cyanosis. Palmar erythema. Facial telangiectases. Blood pressure 130/80 mmHg in the right arm, lying. Pulse 90/minute, regular. JVP + 8 cm. Well healed midline sternotomy scar. Apex displaced to the sixth intercostal space in the anterior axillary line. Ejection click at the base, with a grade 3/6 midsystolic ejection murmur poorly conducted to carotids, and a soft early diastolic decrescendo murmur at the left sternal edge. 6 cm of smooth non-tender hepatomegaly. No splenomegaly. Expiratory wheeze in both lungs.

INITIAL INVESTIGATIONS

Urea 4.6 mmol/l, Na 133 mmol/l, K 3.4 mmol/l, ALT 74 U/l, AST 51 U/l, LDH 430 U/l.

QUESTIONS

1. What is your differential diagnosis?

2. What three non-biochemical investigations, in addition to the ECG, will most help to clarify the diagnosis?

3. Later that evening the patient becomes very aggressive towards fellow-patients and nursing staff. What explanations would you consider likely?

Multiple choice questions

4. The following are appropriate forms of management for patients with the sick sinus syndrome:

(a) *amiodarone*

(b) *rate programmable atrial pacemaker*

(c) *digoxin*

(d) *digoxin plus ventricular pacemaker*

(e) *fixed rate ventricular pacemaker*

5. In Raynaud's phenomenon:

(a) *a family history is uncommon*

(b) *ulceration or infarction of the digits never occurs in the primary form of the condition*

(c) *lumbar sympathectomy may be of prolonged benefit*

(d) *subcutaneous calcification of the fingers may be an associated finding*

(e) *wearing gloves is an important feature of management.*

6. In the management of frostbite:

(a) *early amputation of the gangrenous tissue is desirable*

(b) *heating of the abdomen may improve digital perfusion in the feet*

(c) *oral isosorbide is desirable therapy*

(d) *dextran infusions may be helpful*

(e) *aggressive behaviour should alert the clinician to the likelihood of incipient delirium tremens.*

7. Important risk factors for arteriosclerosis obliterans include:

(a) *diabetes mellitus*

(b) *hyperthyroidism*

(c) *diuretic therapy*

(d) *cigarette smoking*

(e) *arterial hypertension.*

8. Valuable treatment in arteriosclerosis obliterans includes:

(a) *sympathectomy for patients with stable claudication*

(b) *nifedipine*

(c) *regular alcohol*

(d) *regular exercise*

(e) *no smoking.*

ANSWERS AND DISCUSSION

PATIENT 28

1. (a) Ischaemic heart disease in a patient with coincidental valvular heart disease and previous coronary artery surgery.
   (b) Ischaemic heart disease secondary to a stenosing aortic xenograft — the ejection click makes this unlikely.
   (c) Since the murmur is not well conducted to the carotids it may be arising from the pulmonary valve in a patient who has undergone previous pulmonary valvotomy but who has gross right ventricular hypertrophy with or without abnormal coronary vessels supplying the right ventricle.
   (d) Alcoholic liver disease and cardiomyopathy are unlikely to explain the patient's characteristic symptoms or the murmurs.

2. Chest X–ray
   Echocardiogram
   Pyrophosphate scan.

3. Likely explanations:
      alcohol withdrawal syndrome.
      cerebral hypoxia resulting from a low output state — the result of either left or right ventricular dysfunction.
      a respiratory infection may have developed (note wheeze on admission).

4. TRUE   TRUE   TRUE   TRUE   FALSE

The sick sinus syndrome has many variants. The syndrome may be predominantly bradycardic or tachycardic and it is important to relate the patient's symptoms to the relevant arrhythmia, and direct treatment against that arrhythmia. Where bradycardia is symptomatic a demand pacemaker is indicated, where tachycardia is symptomatic digoxin or amiodarone are appropriate and where both arrhythmias are symptomatic combined therapy is indicated.

5. FALSE   TRUE   FALSE   TRUE   TRUE

Primary Raynaud's phenomenon occurs characteristically in young women, often there is a family history of the disorder, and simple measures like avoidance of cold and wearing of gloves are all that is required, since the condition never progresses to ulceration or infarction of the digits. Lumbar sympathectomy is not indicated in the primary condition but may be of temporary benefit in the secondary form. In secondary Raynaud's phenomenon digital infection or ischaemia is common, the onset of the condition is usually in older people and among the many causes are the CRST syndrome (calcinosis, Raynaud's, sclerodactylia and telangiectasis) where subcutaneous digital calcification may occur.

6. FALSE   TRUE   FALSE   TRUE   TRUE

Frostbite commonly occurs in vagrants with a history of alcohol abuse, and in the frail elderly. Surgery should be avoided for as long as possible since the deep tissues are usually well preserved. Treatments to improve the circulation — reflex heating of the abdomen, dextran infusions — may be helpful; isosorbide is not.

7. TRUE   FALSE   FALSE   TRUE   TRUE

Important risk factors for severe arteriosclerotic peripheral vascular disease include smoking, arterial hypertension, hypercholesterolaemia, diabetes mellitus and hypothyroidism. Thiazide diuretics certainly cause a slight rise in plasma lipids but this is a minor problem in terms of the disease process.

8. FALSE   FALSE   FALSE   TRUE   TRUE

Surgery may have a place if there is rest pain, if the viability of the limb is threatened or if the claudication is producing severe disability. Lumbar sympathectomy may be of temporary benefit for those patients with uncomfortable cold feet, but is not of benefit in chronic stable claudication. Vasodilators (nifedipine, alcohol) do not improve claudication. Exercise may encourage a collateral circulation to develop around a blocked artery. Cigarette smoking is particularly harmful in peripheral vascular disease and should be stopped.

2
INTERPRETATION

X-RAYS

Answers are on pages 179–183

QUESTIONS

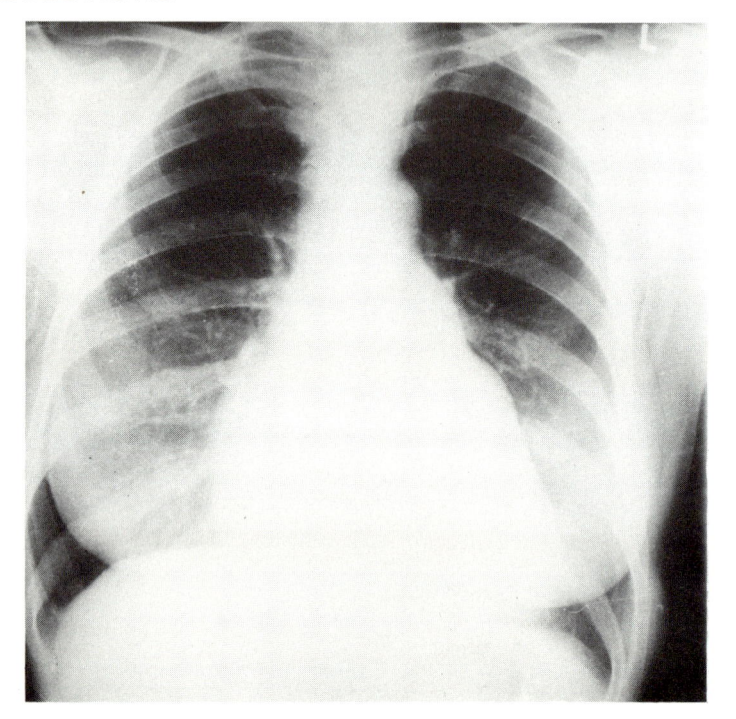

1. Figure 1
A 41 year old mother of two children who is currently undergoing divorce proceedings presents to the cardiology clinic earlier than her appointed annual review complaining of worsening dyspnoea on exertion and sometimes at rest. Her current medication is diazepam 5 mg t.i.d.

(a) *Report her chest X–ray.*

(b) *What other investigations, apart from the ECG which shows sinus rhythm, are indicated?*

(c) *What advice on management should you offer her general practitioner?*

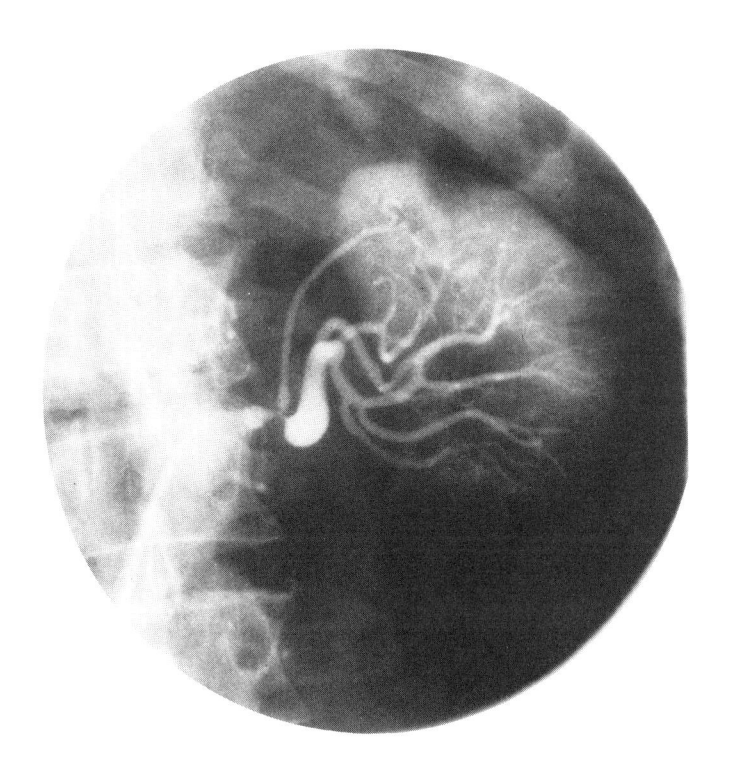

2. Figure 2
A 51 year old joiner who presents to his general practitioner with backache is found to have a blood pressure of 210/130 mmHg. During subsequent inpatient investigation the X–ray presented in Figure 2 is obtained.

(a) *Describe the X-ray appearances.*

(b) *1 week later the patient complains of severe loin pain of sudden onset. What is the differential diagnosis?*

3. Figure 3

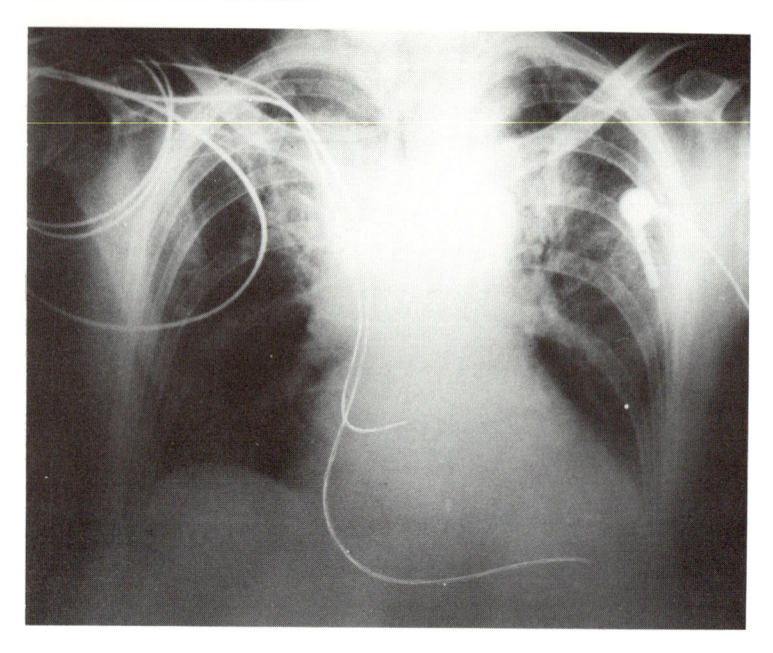

During the management of an acute inferior myocardial infarction complicated by Mobitz Type II block a 73 year old retired schoolmaster has become progressively more hypotensive.

(a) *Report this X–ray.*

(b) *During the 2 hours after this X–ray was taken the patient's blood pressure did not rise. What treatment should now be offered?*

X-RAY INTERPRETATION 167

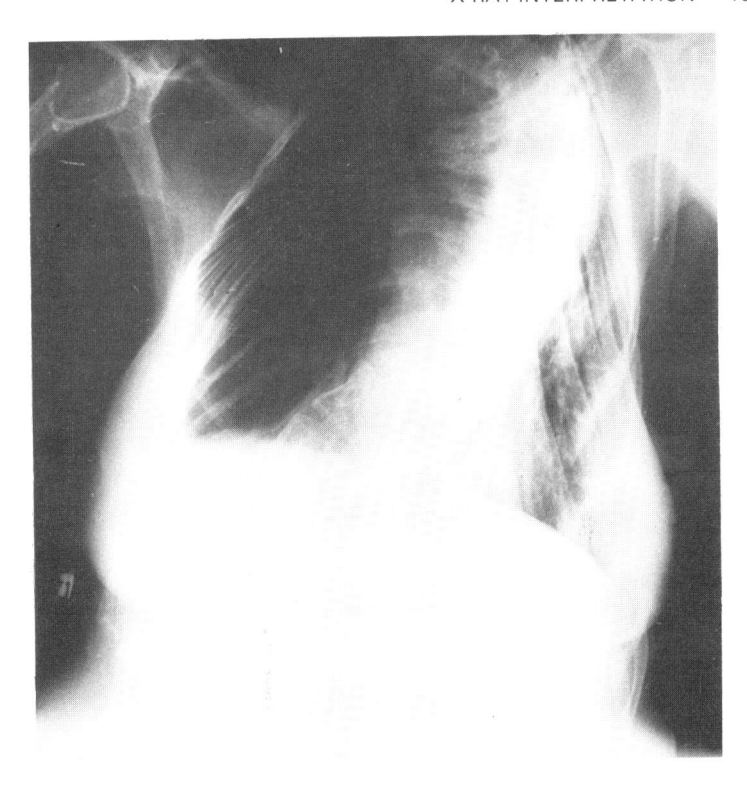

4. Figure 4
   This is the chest X–ray of a 32 year old secretary.

(a) *Describe the X-ray appearances.*

(b) *What ECG abnormalities might you expect to see in this patient?*

5. Figure 5

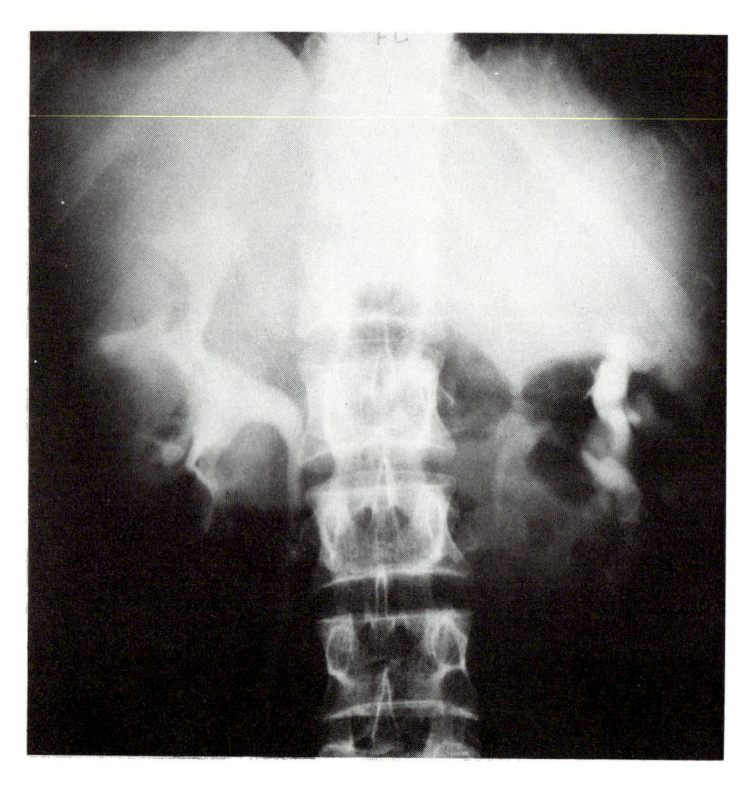

A 36 year old woman whose presenting complaint was of backache has been found to have a blood pressure of 206/126 mmHg. Among her investigations the X-ray of Figure 5 has been obtained.

(a) Describe the appearances.

(b) What is the diagnosis?

(c) Accepting that serum urea and electrolytes are normal, are any other biochemical abnormalities likely?

(d) Are any other members of this patient's family likely to be affected? If so, what is the mode of inheritance?

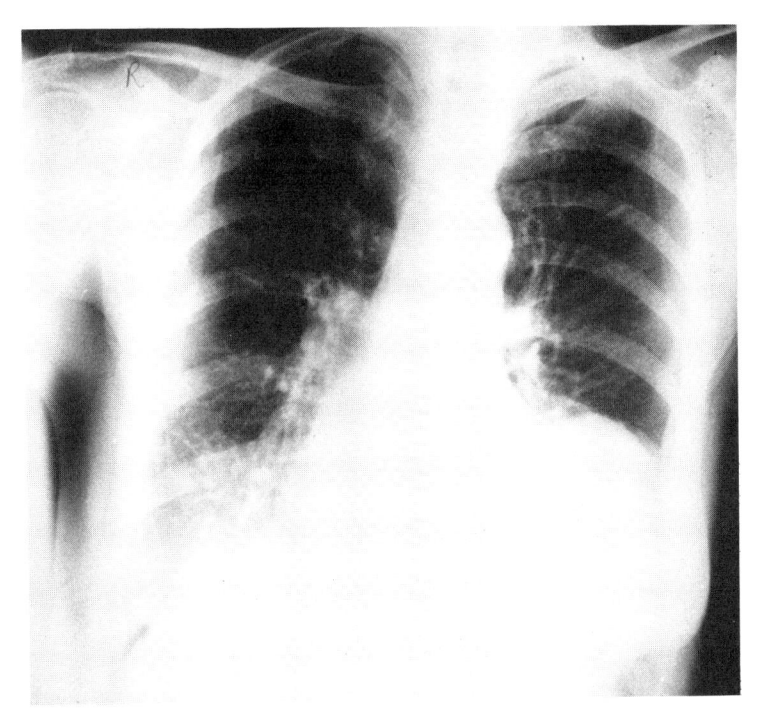

6. Figure 6
A 74 year old woman has presented with chest pain.

(a) *Describe the X-ray appearances.*

(b) *What findings are likely on precordial examination?*

170   CARDIOLOGY REVISION

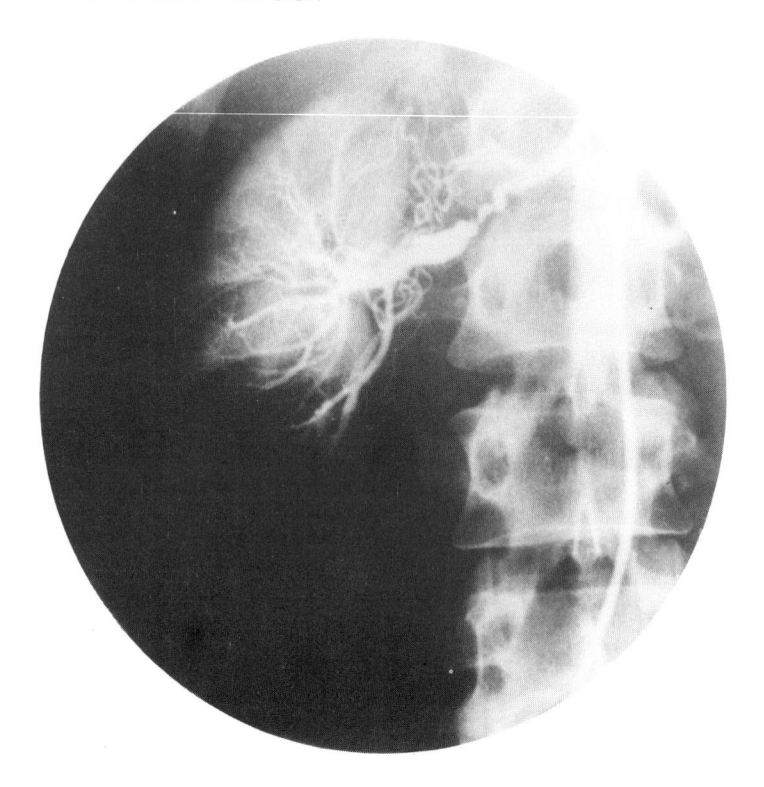

7. Figure 7

The X–ray in Figure 7 has been obtained in a hypertensive 26 year old woman whose presenting complaint is of colicky lower abdominal pain with diarrhoea.

(a) *What does the X–ray show?*

(b) *What is the likely explanation of the abdominal pain?*

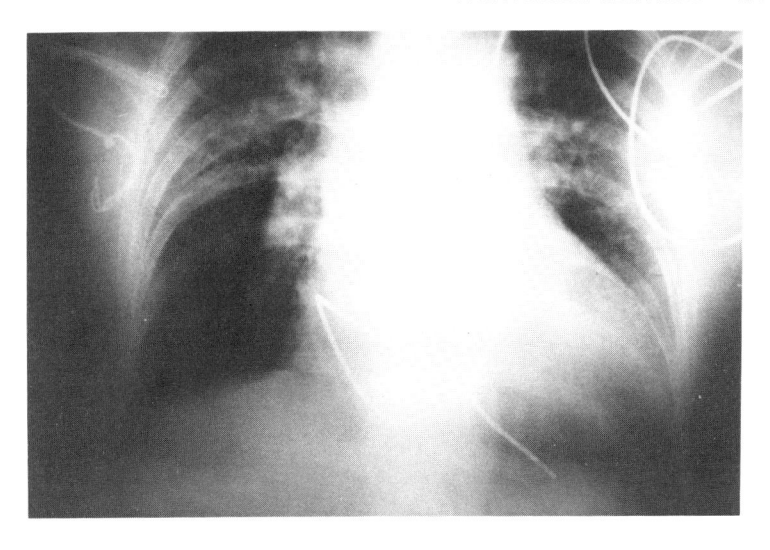

8. Figure 8

Describe the X–ray appearances of this 76 year old woman with the sick sinus syndrome who was admitted with malaise, weight loss and fever.

9. Figure 9

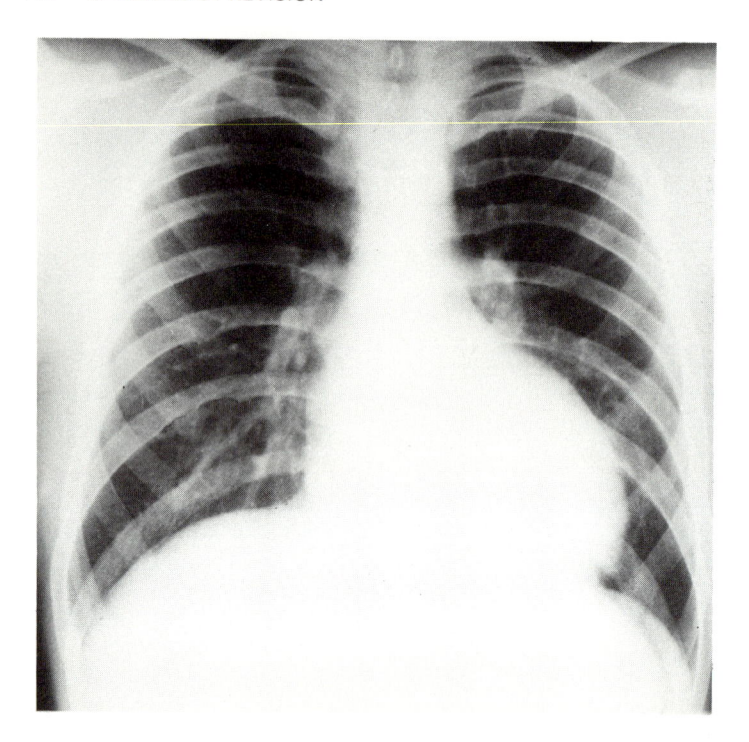

Figure 9 is the chest X-ray of a 19 year old student who has presented with headache and has been found to have a blood pressure of 200/130 mmHg.

(a) *Describe any abnormality you see.*

(b) *Name two clinical signs which it may be useful to identify.*

(c) *What further investigation is indicated?*

(d) *The patient is noted to have a small left pupil. What is the likely explanation of this finding? What further tests, if any, are indicated?*

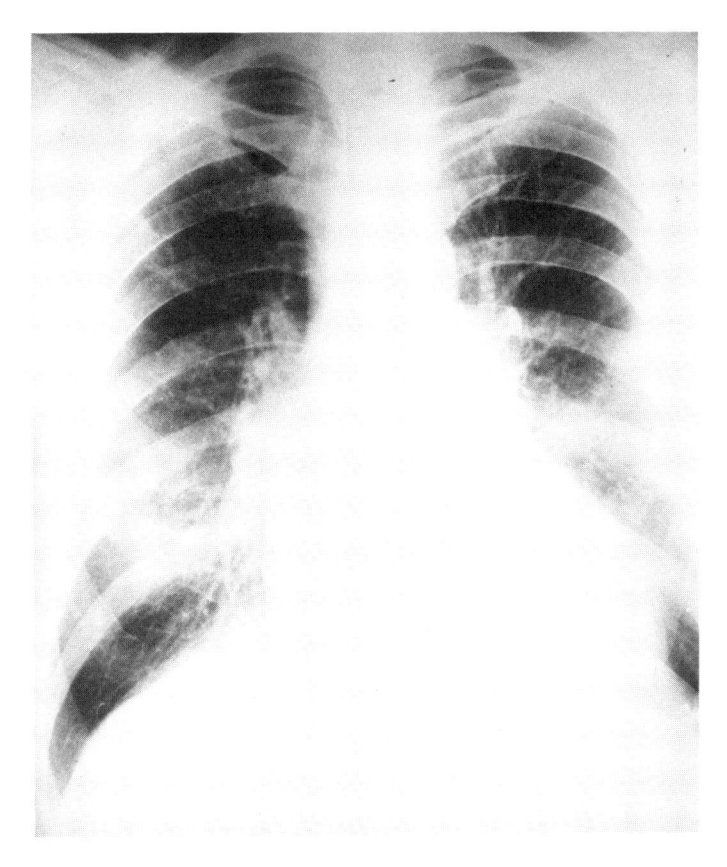

10. Figure 10
A 62 year old insurance agent with longstanding treated hypertension is admitted with a history of visual upset and is found to have a blood pressure of 260/170 mmHg.

(a) *Describe the X-ray appearances.*
(b) *What is the differential diagnosis?*

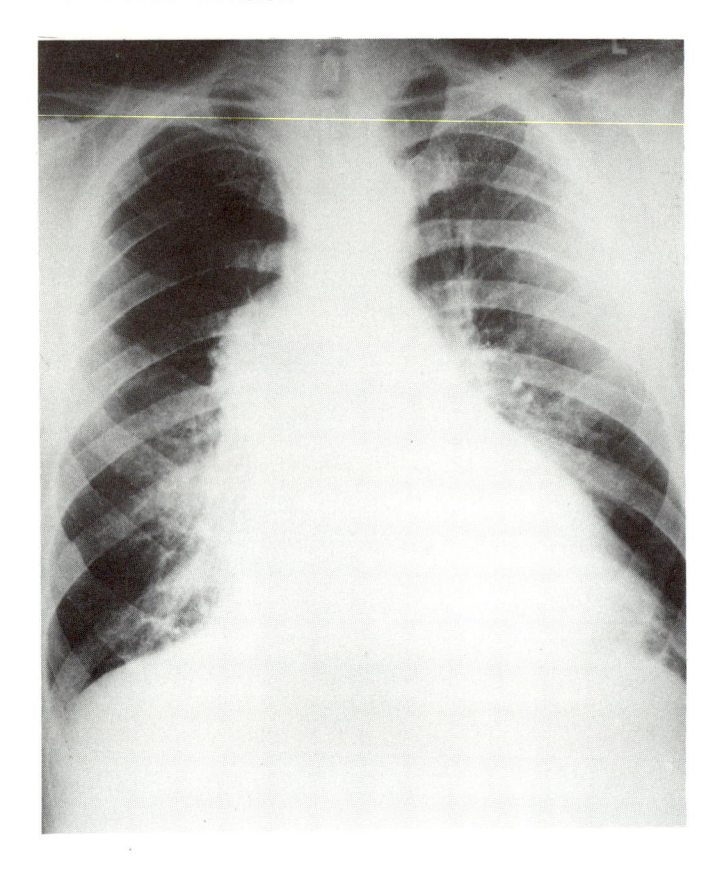

11. Figure 11

This X–ray has been recorded in a 66 year old retired gardener 3 months after cardiac surgery.

(a) *Describe the X–ray appearances.*

(b) *What is the differential diagnosis?*

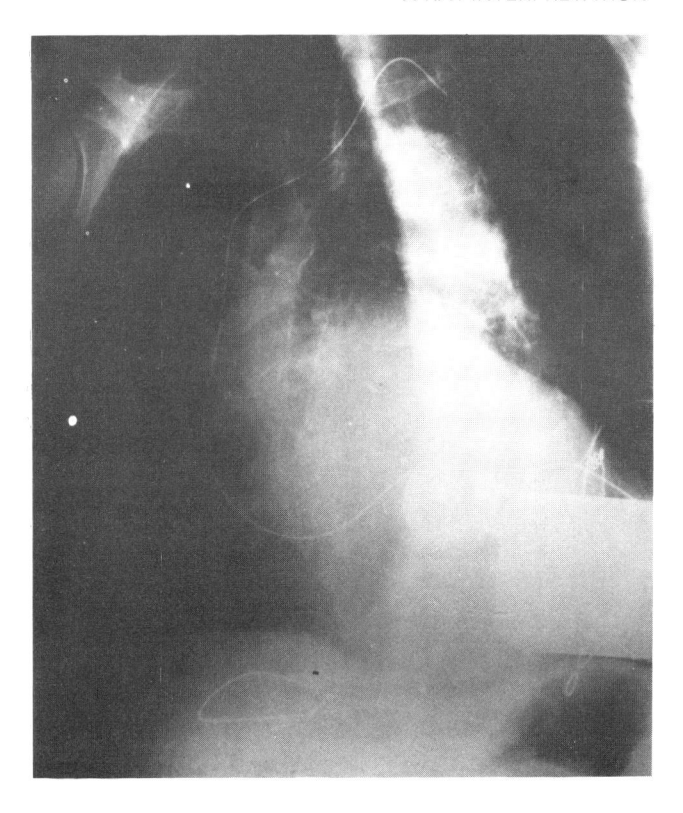

12. Figure 12
This penetrated PA chest film delineates several abnormalities.

(a) *Enumerate the abnormalities.*

(b) *Outline a probable course of events in this patient given the X-ray appearances.*

(c) *Given that the patient has been admitted with nocturnal dyspnoea offer a differential diagnosis.*

13. Figure 13

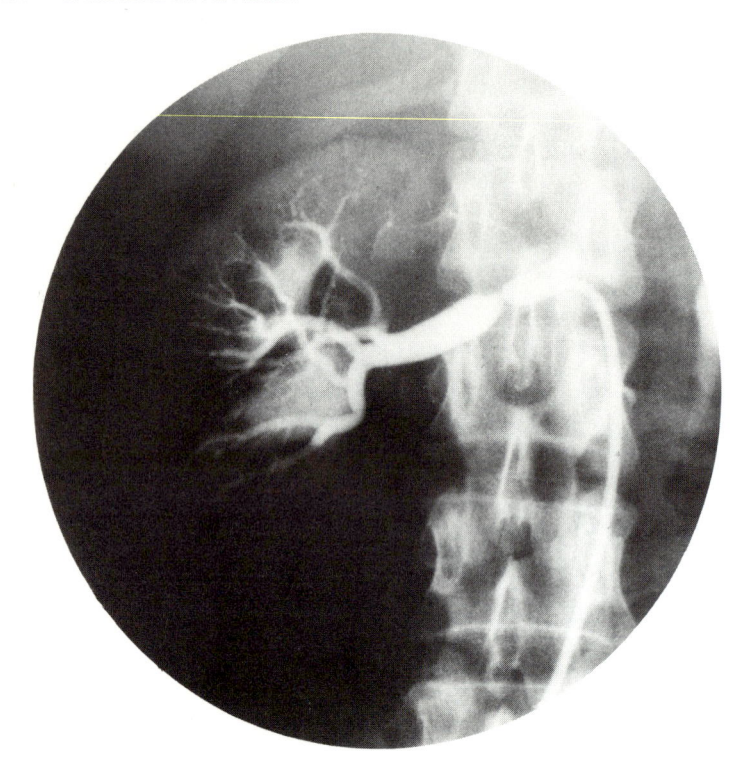

A 25 year old woman is referred for investigation and management from the Family Planning Clinic where a blood pressure of 200/136 mmHg has been recorded. Plasma renin, angiotensin II and aldosterone concentrations are normal, but the X–ray in Figure 13 is obtained.

(a) *Describe the X–ray appearances.*

(b) *Can you draw conclusions on the aetiology of the lesion from the X–ray appearances?*

(c) *What explanation can you offer for the biochemical findings?*

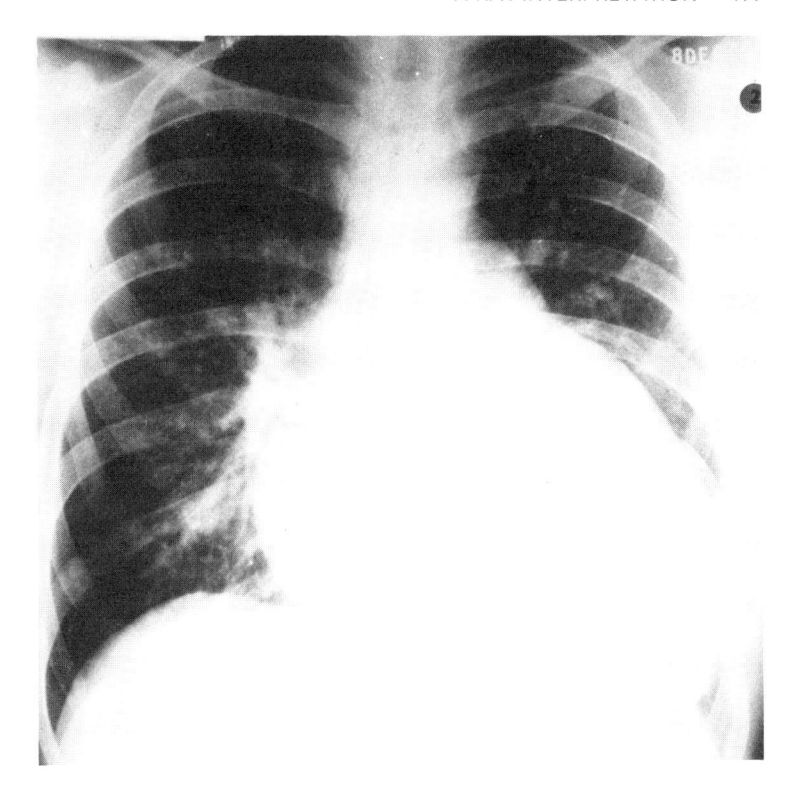

14. Figure 14
This is the X–ray of a 22 year old electrician who has been admitted with a cough productive of yellow spit for 3 days and a 9 year history of exertional dyspnoea.

(a) *Describe the X–ray appearances.*

(b) *What features would you expect on general examination?*

(c) *What is the full blood count likely to show?*

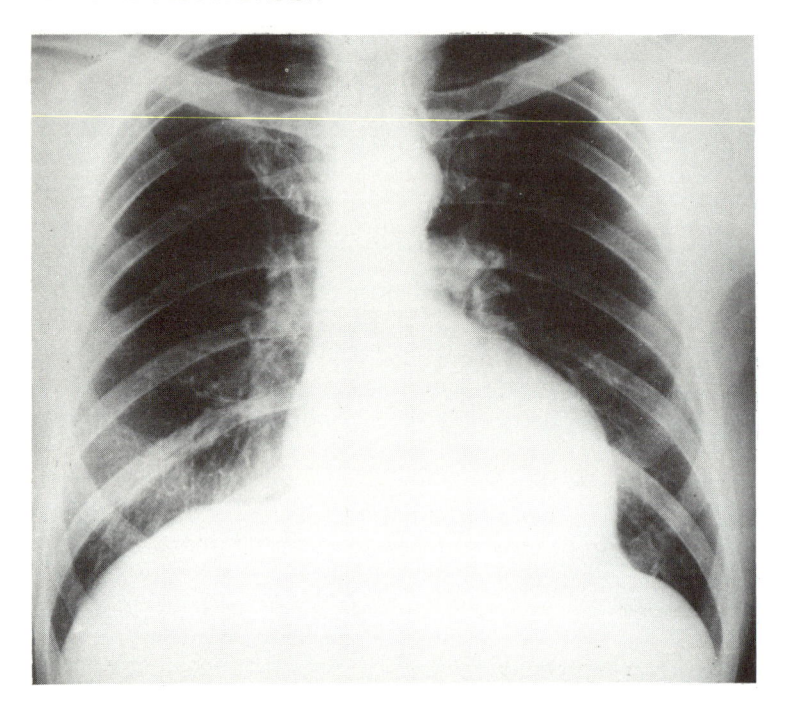

15. Figure 15

A 57 year old lecturer on sabbatical from Turkey attends outpatients complaining of dyspnoea which wakens him at night. He recalls a prolonged episode of indigestion 3 months before, but did not seek medical help at that time. His ECG shows Q waves, ST elevation and T inversion in II, III and aV$_F$.

(a) *Describe the X-ray appearances.*

(b) *What is the differential diagnosis?*

ANSWERS AND DISCUSSION

X-RAYS

1. (a) The X-ray shows cardiomegaly, left atrial prominence, but relatively normal pulmonary vascularity.
   (b) Echocardiography. Venous congestion being minimal, cardiac catheterization is not indicated at present. A 24 hour ambulatory ECG recording will help to exclude paroxysmal atrial fibrillation (intermittent dyspnoea at rest).
   (c) Advise digoxin, diuretic in view of the possible postural character of the dyspnoea, and, given the cardiomegaly, anticoagulation with warfarin.

2. (a) Tight discrete proximal left renal artery stenosis with marked post-stenotic dilatation and with a collateral vessel arising from the stenosed segment and passing to the upper pole of the kidney. Note also early osteophyte formation in lumbar vertebrae.
   (b) i. Occlusion of the left renal artery.
   ii. Rupture of the dilated post-stenotic artery (has there been additional trauma?).
   iii. ? Disc prolapse.

3. (a) This anteroposterior film shows cardiomegaly, pulmonary oedema, temporary atrial and ventricular pacing electrodes passed percutaneously per the right subclavian vein and a cardiac monitor lead.
   (b) Inotropes, e.g. dopamine, may be helpful. The picture is of severe left ventricular dysfunction with a low output state.

4. (a) This shows severe kyphoscoliosis.
   (b) The patient is liable to recurrent respiratory infection with cor pulmonale and equivalent ECG changes of right heart strain. Associated skeletal abnormalities

such as pes cavus or arachnodactyly may indicate that the true diagnosis is Friedrich's ataxia or Marfan's syndrome respectively — each associated with its own ECG abnormalities.

5. (a) This intravenous urogram shows both kidneys to be enlarged with elongation of the pelves, flattened calyces, and indentations due to cysts.
   (b) Polycystic kidney disease.
   (c) Rarely derangement of liver function tests or elevated serum amylase may indicate cysts in the liver and pancreas.
   (d) Other members of this patient's family are likely to be affected since the mode of inheritance in this adult form of polycystic kidney disease is through an autosomal dominant gene with a high degree of penetrance (virtually complete penetrance if the patients survive into the ninth decade).

6. (a) The X–ray shows a bulge on the left ventricular border diagnostic of cardiac aneurysm, cardiomegaly, calcification in the aortic knuckle and pulmonary venous congestion.
   (b) Visible diffuse praecordial pulsation, a palpable diffuse dyskinetic thrust, third or fourth heart sounds, and perhaps accompanying mitral regurgitation murmur.

7. (a) Fibromuscular hyperplasia of the right renal artery — typical 'string of beads' appearances in this right selective renal angiogram with an early collateral circulation via the inferior adrenal vessels.
   (b) Fibromuscular changes in the mesenteric vessels is a likely cause of ischaemic colitis in this patient.

8. The most striking feature is a temporary pacemaker electrode passing down through a persisting left superior vena cava, along the coronary sinus to the right atrium and through the tricuspid valve to the right ventricular apex — a feat of navigation which surprised even the operator! The patient also has cardiomegaly, and the

X-ray marker in swabs over the right pectoral region is visible. The appearances and history suggest that an infected permanent pacemaker has been removed and replaced temporarily by the electrode that is visible. However a chest infection may more simply explain the pyrexial illness.

9. (a) There is notching of the under-surfaces of the ribs, particularly the right 8th and 9th ribs. The appearances are suggestive of a collateral circulation secondary to coarctation of the aorta.
   (b) Delay in the femoral pulses with reduced blood pressure in the legs. Palpable periscapular pulsation from collaterals.
   (c) Aortography; measurement of pressure differences across the coarcted segment; assessment of associated anomalies such as a bicuspid aortic valve, mitral regurgitation, ventricular septal defect and ductus arteriosus by echocardiography and cardiac catheterisation.
   (d) ? Expanding berry aneurysm. Computerized tomography of the head, and four-vessel angiography may be indicated. Berry aneurysms are a further common anomaly in patients with coarctation and many adults with coarctation die following intracranial haemorrhage.

10. (a) Cardiomegaly, left ventricular enlargement, interstitial and alveolar pulmonary oedema.
    (b) i. Beta blocker effects with sympathetic stimulation due to pulmonary oedema.
       ii. Clonidine withdrawal.
       iii. Malignant phase hypertension — has, for instance, renal artery stenosis developed during long-standing essential hypertension?
       iv. Myocardial infarction with pain and release of catecholamines.
       v. Subarachnoid haemorrhage with neurogenic pulmonary oedema.
       vi. Non-compliance with medication.

11. (a) Cardiomegaly, left ventricular prominence, rounded bulge of the right heart border at the level of the proximal ascending aorta, and pulmonary venous congestion.
    (b) i. Post-stenotic dilation in aortic stenosis.
        ii. Pseudoaneurysm of ascending aorta following aortic valve surgery.
        iii. Expanding aneurysm of ascending aorta (rule out syphilitic) with cardiomegaly possibly due to aortic regurgitation (unlikely).

12. (a) Starr-Edwards mitral valve prosthesis.
    Pacemaker pulse generator situated low over left chest wall.
    Permanent transvenous pacemaker electrode situated high in the right ventricle.
    Old pacemaker electrode in epigastric position (epicardial electrode).
    Calcified bronchial cartilage.
    Scoliosis.
    (b) Damage (temporary or permanent) to the conducting system at the time of mitral valve replacement has led to an epicardial pacemaker being inserted originally. This has since been replaced by a transvenous system.
    (c) i. Paraprosthetic valve leak.
        ii. Concurrent aortic valve disease.
        iii. Pacemaker malfunction.
        iv. Sick sinus syndrome with paroxysmal atrial fibrillation.
        v. Simply congestive cardiac failure.

13. (a) A tight concentric stenosis at the junction of the proximal and middle thirds of the right main renal artery is present with slight post-stenotic dilatation and a developing collateral vessel via the inferior adrenal artery. Note also the pyelogram in the left kidney (as well as right) from previous contrast injections.
    (b) No. Fibromuscular dysplasia may cause a single discrete stenosis as well as atheroma or extrinsic pressure. Given this woman's history atheroma would be unlikely.

(c) Renin, angiotensin II and aldosterone levels initially elevated may return to normal when a stenosis has been present for some time. Angiotensin is thought to have slow pressor effects (in addition to its immediate pressor activity) which are potent even with plasma levels within the normal range.

14. (a) The appearances are of gross cardiomegaly, with possibly some patchy opacification at the right base but otherwise clear lung fields.
(b) Given the prolonged history and the gross cardiac enlargement, congenital heart disease is one possibility with peripheral cyanosis and finger clubbing. Ebstein's anomaly and a dilated cardiomyopathy are other possibilities with accompanying signs of right heart failure.
(c) Polycythaemia, plus possible leucocytosis from chest infection.

15. (a) The appearance is of left ventricular dilatation with a smooth if abnormal left ventricular contour. There is also some calcification in the aortic knuckle.
(b) The ECG findings taken in conjunction with the X–ray suggest left ventricular aneurysm, though the X–ray appearances may be due simply to a dilated poorly functioning ventricle with the ECG indicative of more recent infarction.

ECG

Answers are on pages 201–206

QUESTIONS

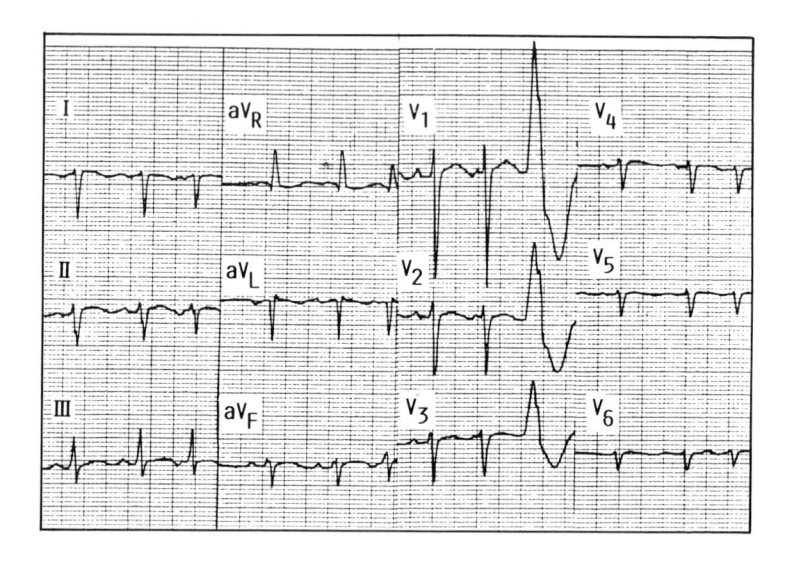

1. Figure 16
Study this ECG obtained from a patient who has been admitted to the surgical wards for investigation of persistent diarrhoea.

(a) *What abnormalities are present?*

(b) *Which simple manoeuvre will clarify the diagnosis?*

(c) *What advice would you offer?*

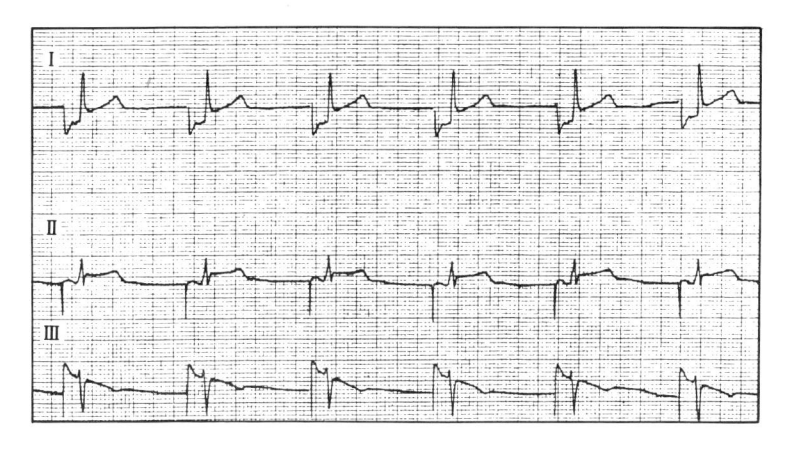

2. Figure 17
Report this ECG.

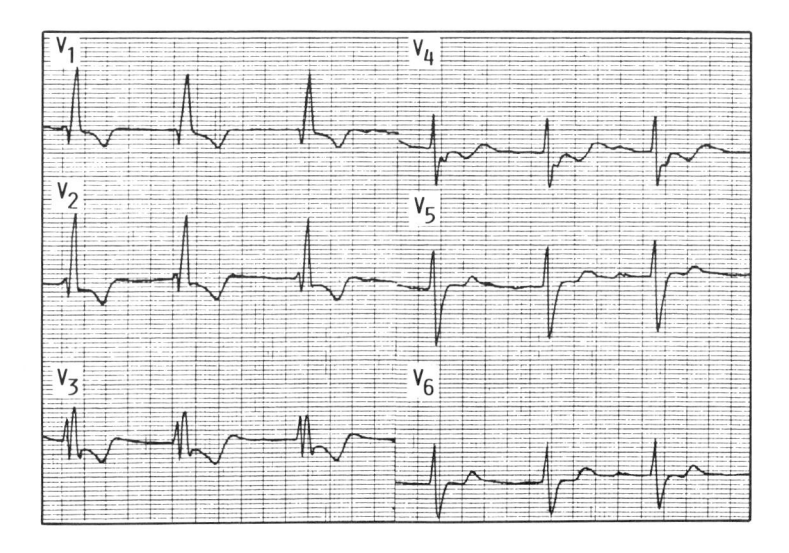

3. Figure 18
Report this ECG of a 55 year old lawyer who has been admitted with chest pain.

4. Figure 19

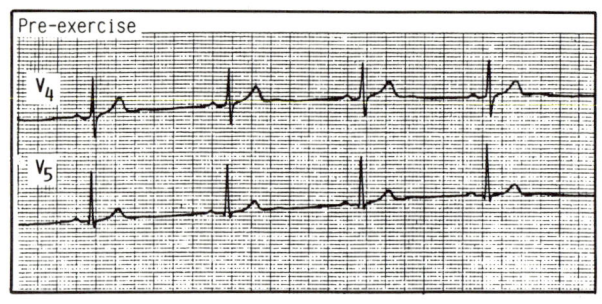

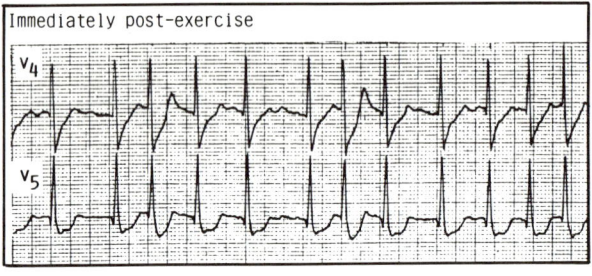

A 52 year old Sikh shopkeeper presents to the cardiology clinic 3 months after coronary artery bypass graft surgery with left shoulder discomfort in the mornings. Describe any abnormalities on these recordings.

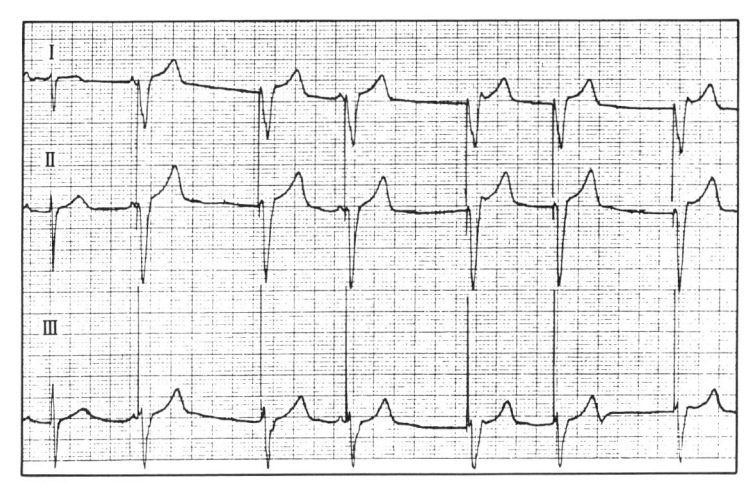

5. Figure 20
This ECG has been recorded in the accident and emergency department in a patient whom the staff nurse tells you is in atrial fibrillation.

(a) *Report this ECG.*

(b) *What treatment do you advise?*

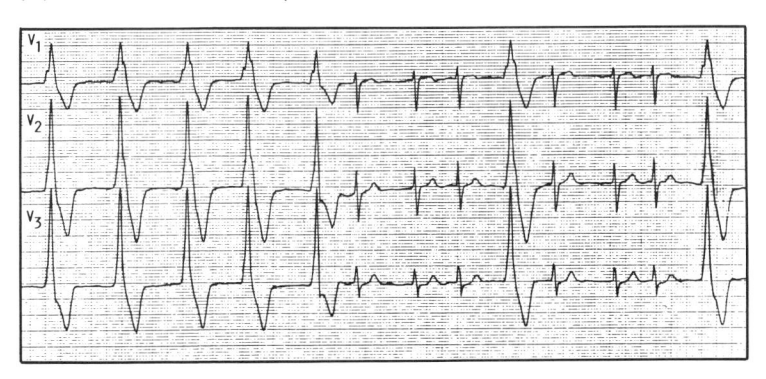

6. Figure 21
A 59 year old nurse presents with deteriorating palpitation and nausea.

(a) *Report this ECG.*

(b) *What is the differential diagnosis?*

(c) *What is the treatment of choice?*

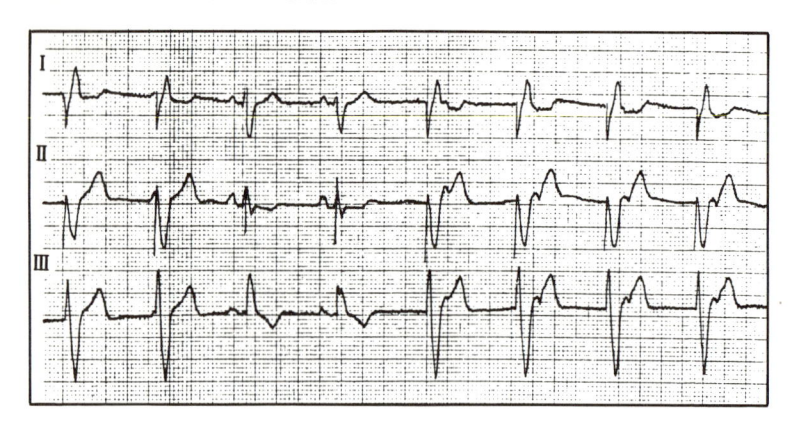

7. Figure 22

This ECG has been recorded in a patient who complains bitterly of palpitation at night.

(a) Report this ECG.

(b) What is the likely cause of the palpitation?

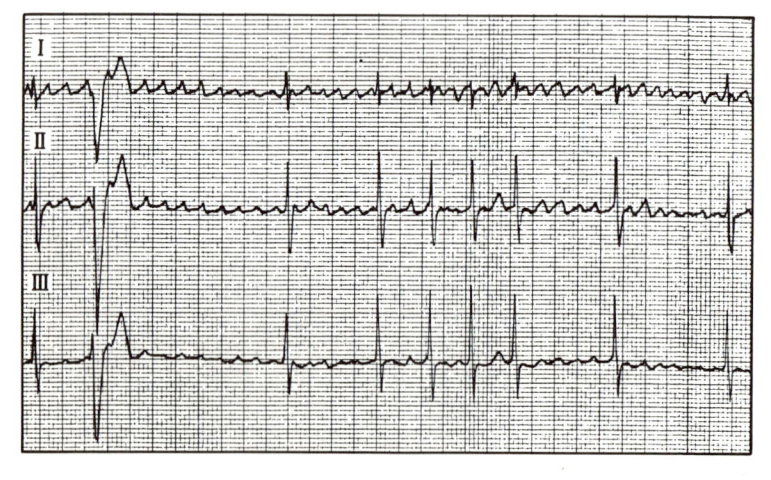

8. Figure 23

This recording has been made in a 52 year old woman who one month previously underwent closed mitral valvotomy.

(a) Report this ECG.

(b) What is the treatment of choice?

ELECTROCARDIOGRAM INTERPRETATION 189

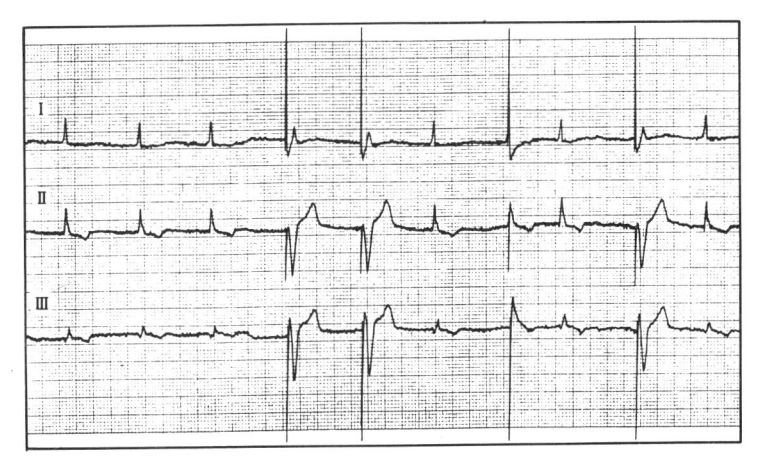

9. Figure 24
73 year old miner complains of dizzy spells. He is on no medication and otherwise enjoys good health.

(a) *Report this ECG.*

(b) *Describe any therapeutic interventions which you think are desirable.*

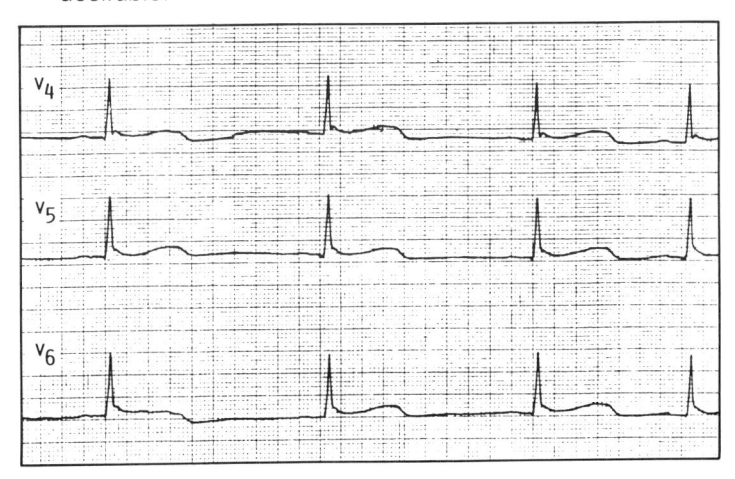

10. Figure 25
(a) *What abnormalities are present on this trace (Figure 25)?*

(b) *Which class of drugs is most likely to have produced this picture?*

(c) *Which drugs, if any, are indicated in the emergency management of this patient?*

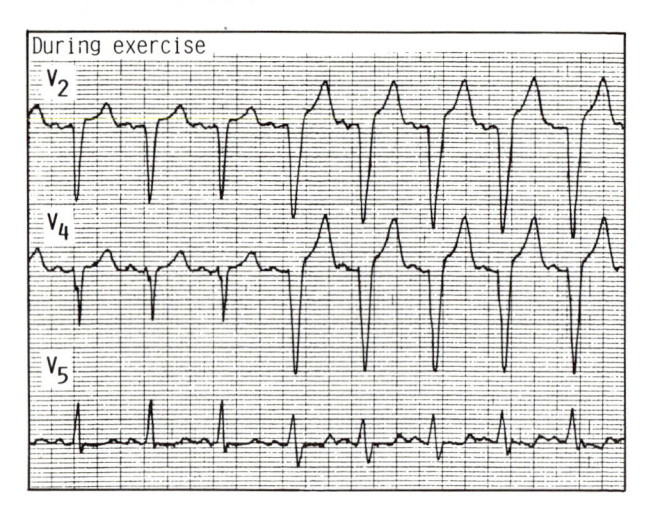

11. Figure 26
(a) *Describe this recording obtained during gentle asymptomatic treadmill testing.*

(b) *What action, if any, should be taken?*

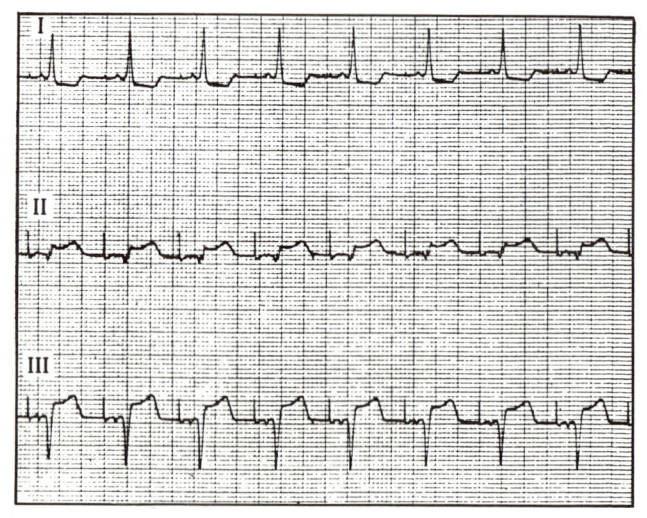

12. Figure 27
A 52 year old housewife presents with severe indigestion, nausea and lightheadedness and is admitted to the medical ward.

What does this ECG, recorded on the morning after admission, show?

13. Figure 28

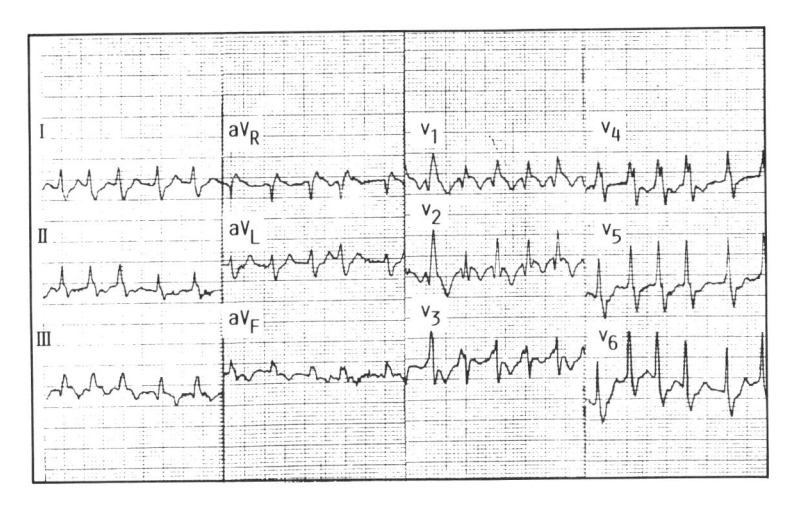

A 62 year old hotelier with Wegener's granulomatosis has collapsed in the ward 3 days after the commencement of prednisolone and azathioprine.

(a) *Report this ECG.*

(b) *What is the likely explanation for the patient's collapse?*

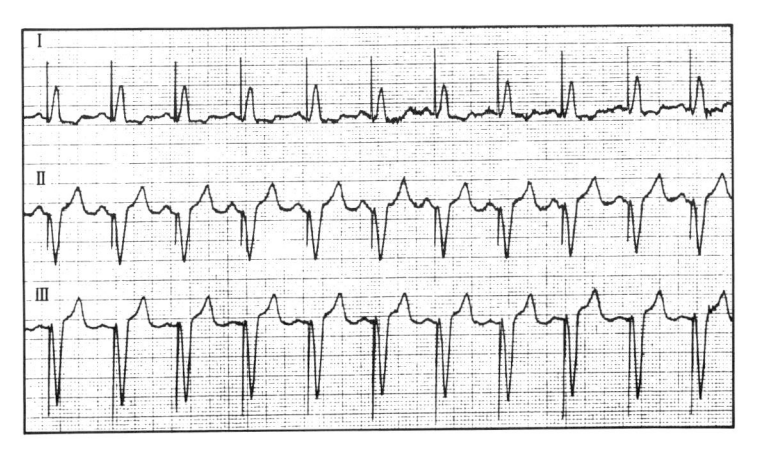

14. Figure 29

(a) *Describe this ECG.*

(b) *What is the diagnosis?*

15. Figure 30

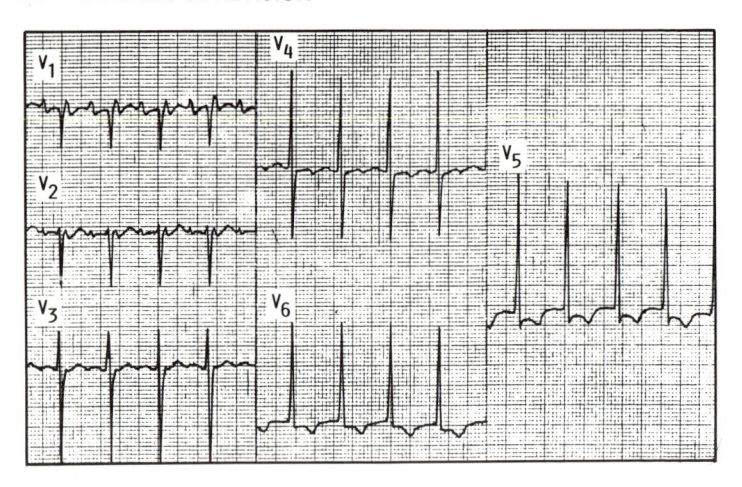

(a) What abnormalities are present on this ECG?

(b) In the further management of this patient, what is likely to be the drug of choice? Explain your choice.

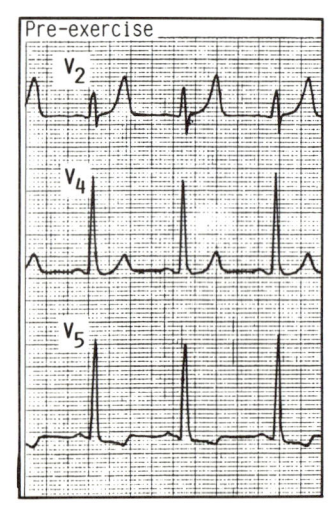

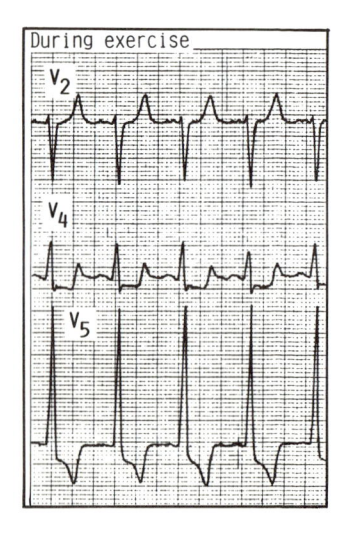

16. Figure 31

This recording has been made in a 48 year old welder who, after an inferior myocardial infarction four weeks previously, is due to start a rehabilitation exercise programme.

Describe how you would manage this patient, and explain your mode of management.

ELECTROCARDIOGRAM INTERPRETATION   193

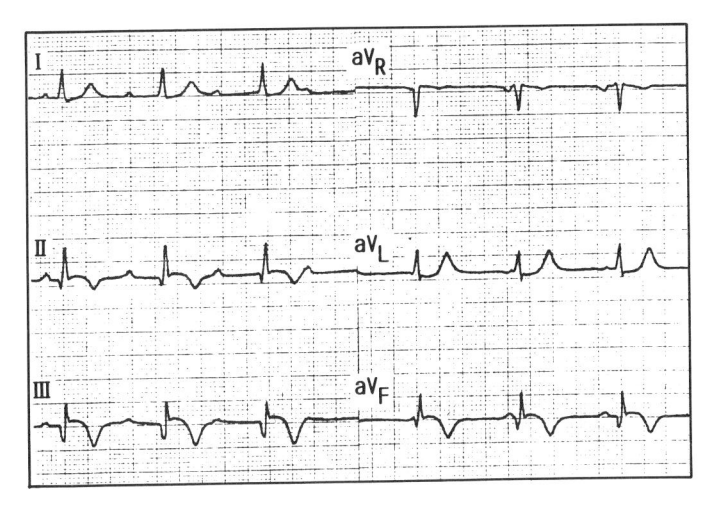

17. Figure 32
(a) Report this ECG.
(b) What is the treatment of choice?
(c) What is the likely prognosis?

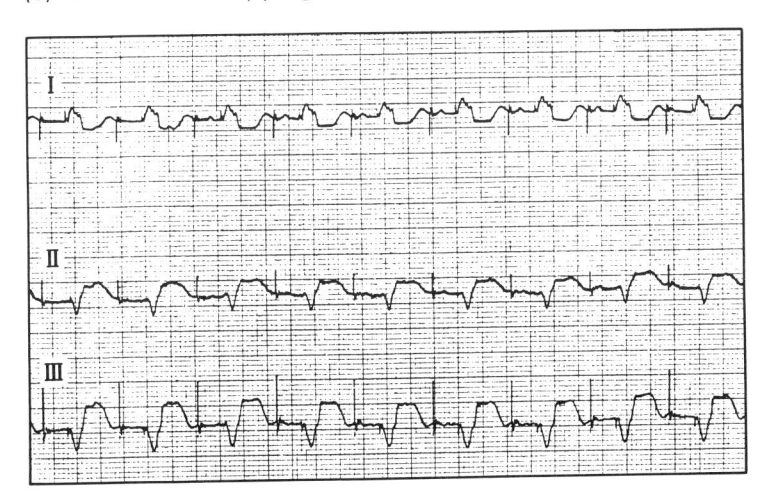

18. Figure 33
(a) Report this ECG.
(b) From which problem do you think the patient suffers?

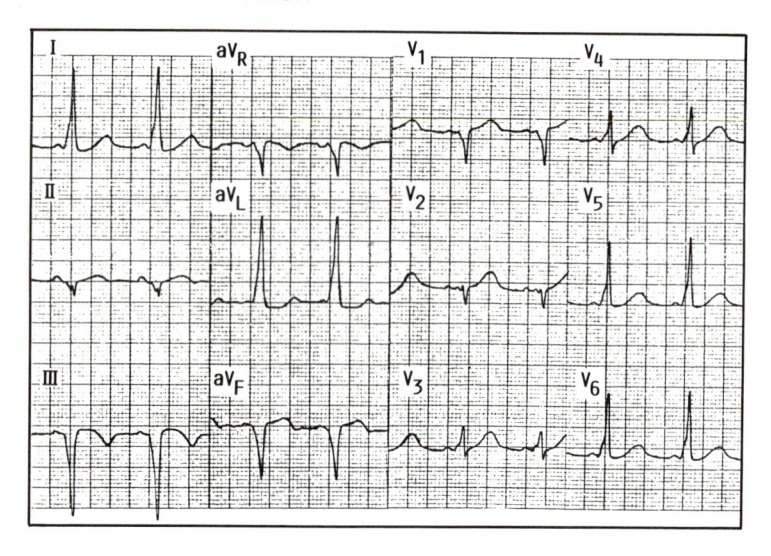

19. Figure 34
Report this ECG.

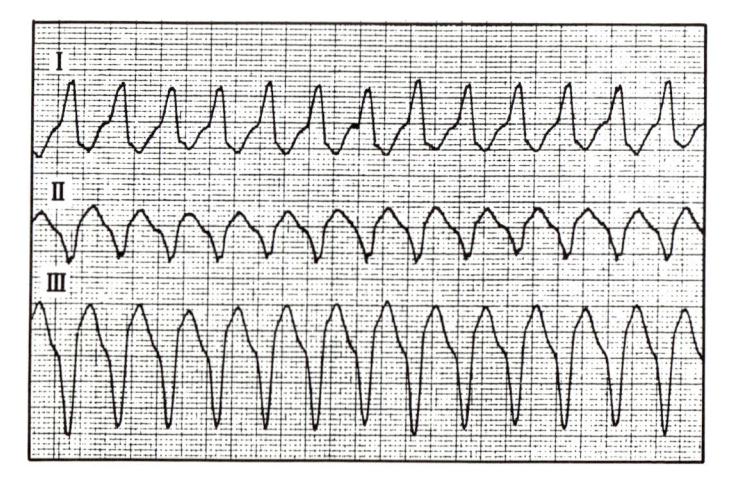

20. Figure 35
(a) *Report this ECG.*
(b) *Outline how you would manage this patient.*

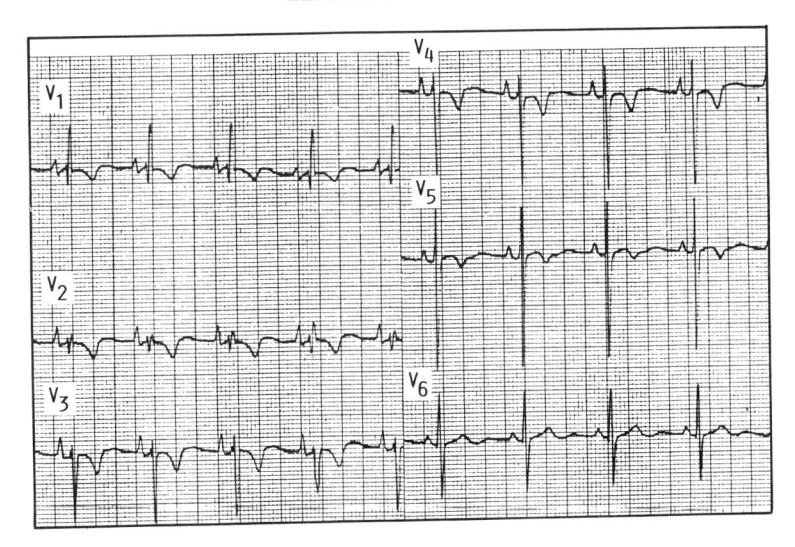

21. Figure 36
(a) *Report this ECG.*
(b) *With which symptoms is the patient likely to have presented?*

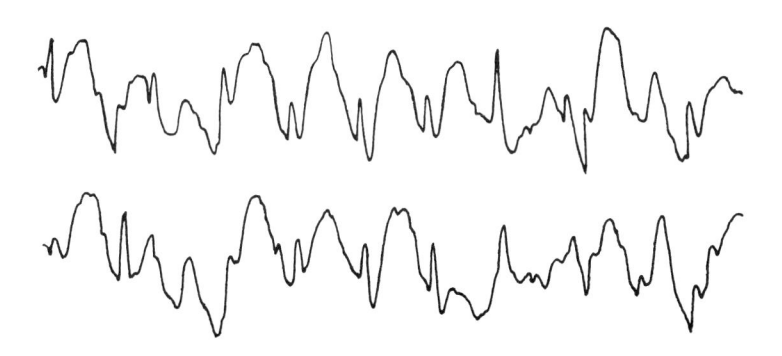

22. Figure 37
This trace has been obtained from a 23 year old typist who complains of paroxysmal dizziness and palpitation.
Report this trace.

23. Figure 38

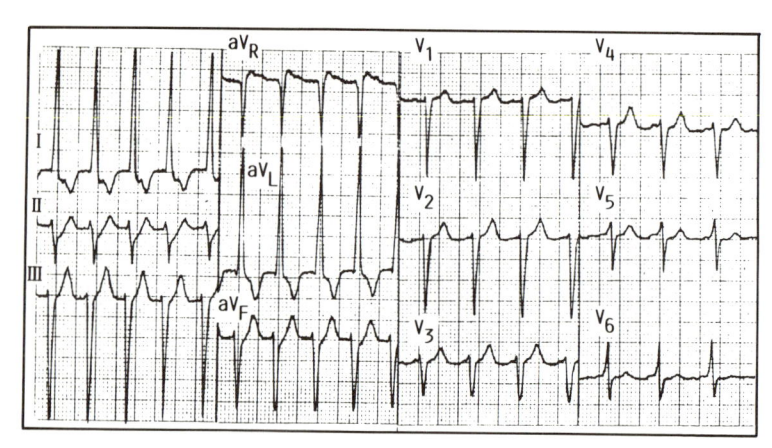

This recording has been made in a 58 year old woman who has presented with biliary colic.

(a) Report this ECG.

(b) What biochemical test(s) would you wish to perform after reviewing this ECG?

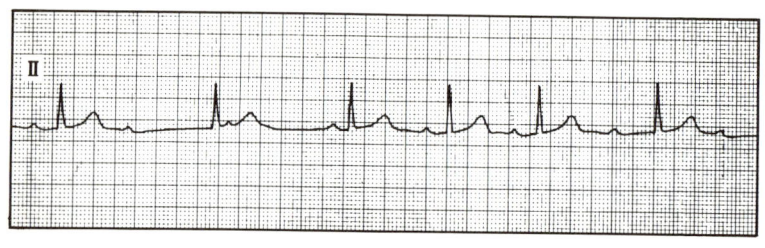

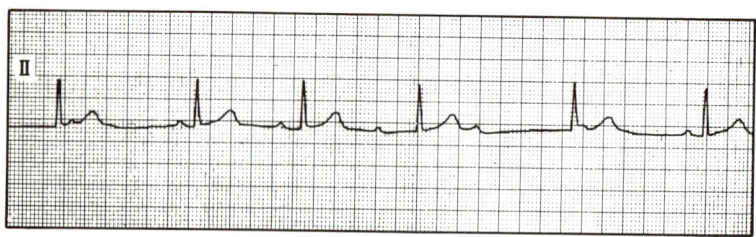

24. Figure 39

This is part of the 24 hour ambulatory ECG recording of a young epileptic patient.

(a) What is the ECG diagnosis?

(b) What is the treatment for this problem?

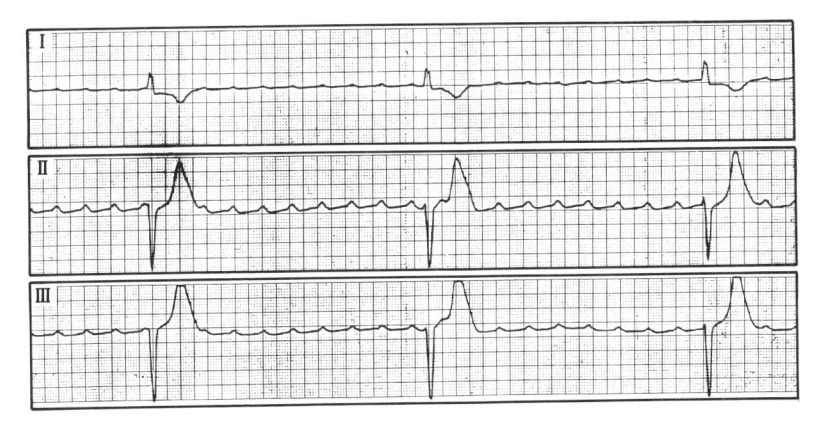

25. Figure 40
(a) Report this ECG.
(b) Of what symptoms is the patient likely to complain?

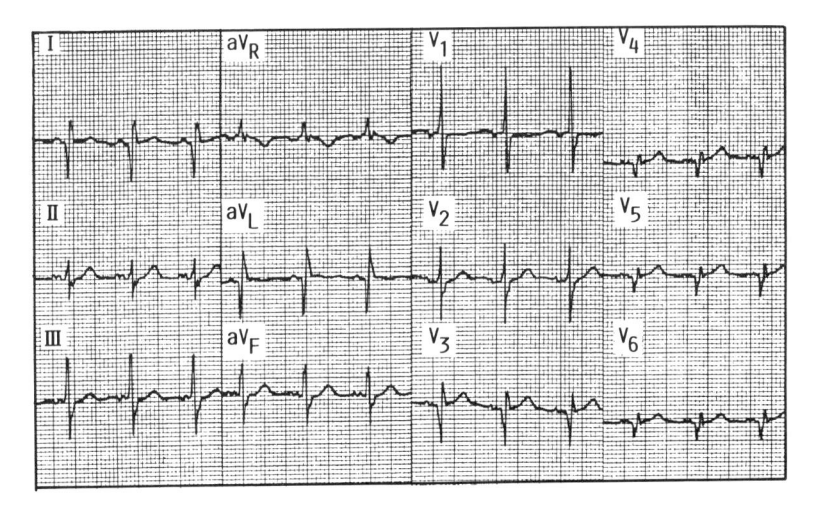

26. Figure 41
Report this ECG of a 47 year old teacher who has presented with exertional dyspnoea.

27. Figure 42

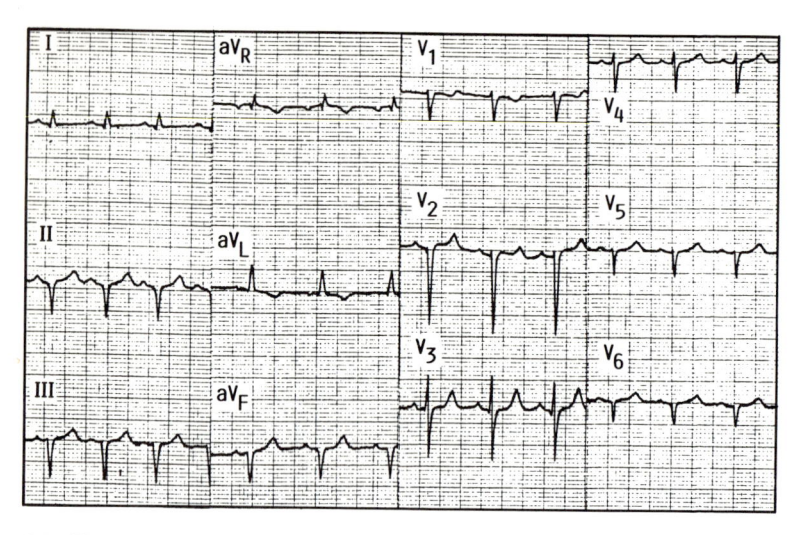

(a) *Report this ECG.*

(b) *What is/are the likely explanation(s) for this recording?*

28. Figure 43

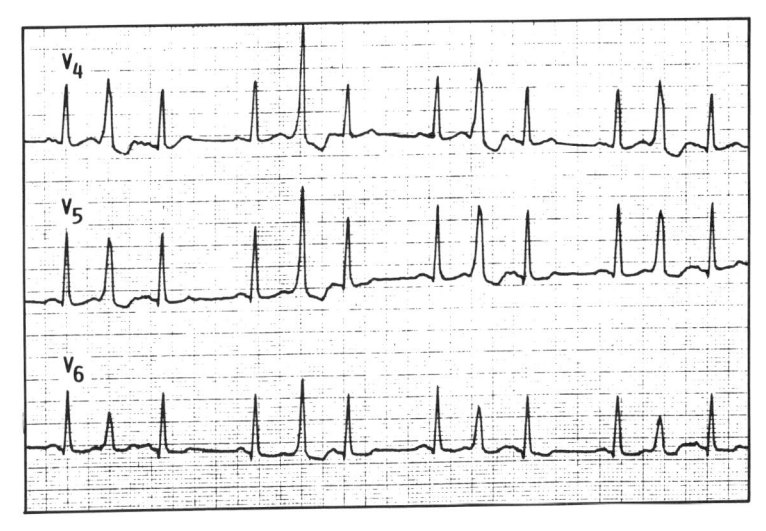

This ECG has been recorded in a 36 year old plumber who has presented with abdominal pain and in whom the following results have been obtained:

Hb 11.2 g/dl   6% reticulocytes

Plasma results: urea 2.6 mmol/l, sodium 124 mmol/l potassium 2.8 mmol/l, ALT 190 U/l.

(a) *Report the ECG.*
(b) *What is the likely diagnosis?*

200 CARDIOLOGY REVISION

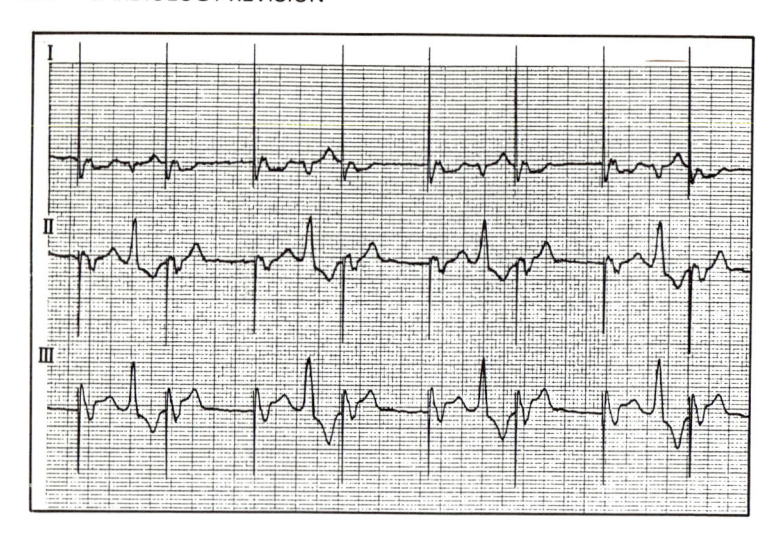

29. Figure 44
Report this ECG.

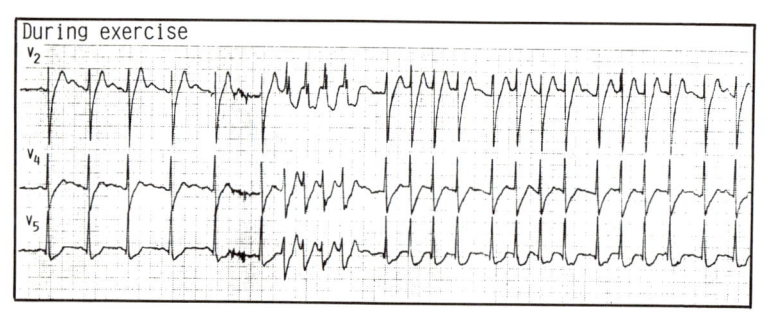

30. Figure 45
(a) Describe abnormal features on this ECG trace.
(b) What significance do you attribute to these features?

ANSWERS AND DISCUSSION

ECG

1. (a) Inverted P waves in I suggesting dextrocardia. Supraventricular and ventricular ectopics. The apparent rotation may be explained by dextrocardia also.
   (b) Chest examination: Transposition of the ECG leads as illustrated (fig. 46).

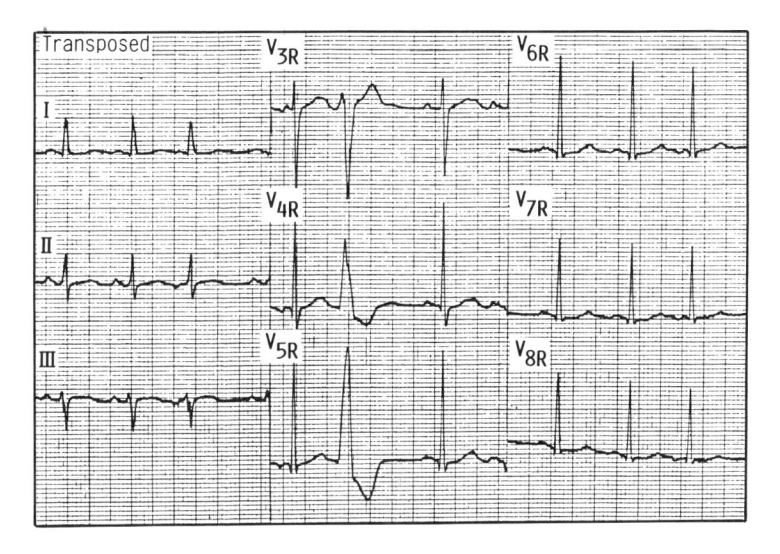

   (c) To the surgeon — beware of the direction in which the sigmoidoscope is passed — the patient may have situs inversus.

2. This shows a normally functioning atrial pacemaker at 50 beats per minute.

3. Complete right bundle branch block: atrial fibrillation.

4. Post-exercise the patient's rhythm has changed to atrial fibrillation and ST segments are depressed by 3 mm — each factor would constitute a positive exercise test in its own right.

5. (a) This trace shows a malfunctioning ventricular pacemaker — being inhibited intermittently by the T wave of the preceding paced beat, producing an unusual form of bigeminy.
   (b) Replacement of the pulse generator if the system is a simple one; increasing the sensing threshold if a programmable pacemaker is in situ.

6. (a) Idioventricular rhythm changing to atrial fibrillation with ventricular ectopics.
   (b) Digoxin toxicity: myocardial ischaemia.
   (c) Withdraw digoxin if appropriate.
   Expectant treatment.
   Beta blockade may be necessary.

7. (a) Normal right ventricular pacemaker function at c̄ 72/min with fusion beats.
   (b) These fusion beats are a possible explanation for the palpitation.

8. (a) Atrial flutter/fibrillation (with a controlled ventricular rate) and one ventricular ectopic.
   (b) Continue anticoagulants, temporarily withdraw digoxin, and electively attempt DC cardioversion.

9. (a) Normal right ventricular pacemaker function with underlying atrial fibrillation. The repolarization changes in II and III may be the result of prior pacing or may suggest digoxin effect but the patient is on no medication.
   (b) The dizzy spells may be due to paroxysmal tachyarrhythmias — 24 hour ECG recording will be helpful. Consider non-cardiac causes — ? cervical spondylosis.

10. (a) Severe sinus bradycardia, J waves, prolonged QT intervals.
   (b) Phenothiazines.
   (c) Gradual rewarming of this hypothermic patient is indicated — medication may be hazardous.

11. (a) The patient remains in sinus rhythm but changes from normal conduction to left bundle branch block.
   (b) The test is positive and should be stopped.

12. The patient has had an atrial pacemaker inserted, and the underlying ventricular complexes show an inferior myocardial infarction with 'reciprocal' changes in I.

13. (a) Atrial fibrillation with a very rapid ventricular rate; marked right bundle branch conduction abnormality.
   (b) Acute pulmonary embolism.

14. (a) Normal P waves are followed by a pacing spike and paced ventricular complexes.
   (b) Characteristic of a VAT pacemaker (Ventricle paced; Atrium sensed; mode of response Triggered).

15. (a) Atrial tachycardia with 2:1 block.
   Left ventricular hypertrophy and strain.
   (b) Beta blockade will be both antihypertensive and prophylactic against recurrence of the arrhythmia (assuming LVH is due to hypertension).

16. This exercise test is positive in leads other than inferior leads, and suggests disease in coronary arteries other than the right coronary artery. This patient requires coronary angiography and consideration of coronary artery bypass grafting.

17. (a) A-V dissociation; changes of acute inferior myocardial infarction.
   (b) Temporary pacemaker insertion.
   (c) Since the arrhythmia is part of an acute inferior infarct spontaneous resolution of the arrhythmia is likely.

18. (a) This ECG shows A-V sequential pacing, the ventricular pacing occurring 0.20 seconds after the atrial pacing. There are some atrial fusion beats. The paced rate is approximately 95/minute.
    (b) Probable myocardial infarction with conduction defect and systemic hypotension. AV sequential pacing allows retention of the atrial kick which may contribute over 30% of cardiac output in situations of poor ventricular function.

19. The appearances are those of Type B Wolff-Parkinson-White syndrome with a short PR interval, negative delta waves in II, III aV$_F$ simulating the Q waves of myocardial infarction, negative delta waves in V$_{1, 2}$ and tall R waves in the left chest leads, suggesting conduction through an anomalous pathway in the right ventricle.

20. (a) This shows a broad complex tachycardia at 150/minute. Whether the origin is supraventricular or ventricular cannot be established from this trace.
    (b) If the patient is tolerating the arrhythmia poorly then rapid cardioversion is indicated. If the patient is tolerating the tachycardia well, elective cardioversion may be contemplated, but intravenous disopyramide effective against both supraventricular and ventricular arrhythmias may be helpful.

21. (a) Sinus rhythm, right atrial hypertrophy, incomplete right bundle branch block, right ventricular strain pattern.
    (b) If the underlying problem is cardiac then symptoms of right heart failure will predominate — ankle swelling, abdominal discomfort, jaundice — whereas if the primary problem is respiratory the dyspnoea, cough and wheeze of airways disease will be dominant.

22. Don't be deceived. This EEG trace shows the characteristic spike and wave discharge of petit mal epilepsy.

23. (a) Sinus tachycardia at 150/min slowing to 110/min by the time the chest leads are recorded; left axis devia-

tion; voltage criteria for left ventricular hypertrophy and strain (R in I and aV$_L$ = 30 mm).
(b) Serum urea and creatinine (and electrolytes) to assess end-organ damage elsewhere. More extensive biochemical testing — urinary normetadrenaline levels, etc. — may be indicated depending on the patient's history and other clinical findings (an alternative cause for LVH must be considered).

24. (a) Wenckebach Type II A-V block.
(b) During sleep this may occur occasionally in normal individuals. Plasma anticonvulsant levels should be estimated since carbamazepine in particular may precipitate block. Unless the arrhythmia correlates with symptoms it does not call for action in its own right.

25. (a) AV dissociation with a very, very slow ventricular rate.
(b) It is possible that the patient would be unconscious at this slow ventricular rate though patients with surprisingly slow rates may be discovered incidentally. Assuming this is an intermittent problem the patient may complain of dizziness or fainting attacks or typical symptoms of Stokes-Adams attacks.

26. Sinus rhythm; the bifid P wave in II is within normal limits; PR = 0.12 sec; Q in I, V$_{3-6}$ with isoelectric ST segments and upright T wave; tall R in V$_1$V$_2$. The appearances are compatible with posterior extension of an established lateral myocardial infarction.

27. (a) Sinus rhythm; left axis deviation; the chest leads all show rS or RS complexes.
(b) Assuming that the leads have been attached in the customary manner chest deformity such as kyphoscoliosis is the likely explanation.

28. (a) This trace shows interpolated ventricular ectopics.
(b) The liver dysfunction, anaemia with reticulocytosis and hyponatraemia (spurious) suggest Zieve's syndrome — the arrhythmia is compatible with alcohol effects on the myocardium.

29. This shows normal right ventricular pacing at c̄ 72/minute with interpolated ventricular ectopics.

30. (a) During exercise sinus rhythm at c̄ 75/min is followed by four broad complex beats with retrograde atrial conduction then by atrial fibrillation with clear plane ST depression in V_5.
(b) This is a positive exercise test, and should prompt further cardiac investigation such as coronary angiography.

DATA

Answers are on pages 212–215

QUESTIONS

1. A 32 year old teacher complains of recurrent central chest discomfort. She has suffered from sore throats for many years but these have been worse lately. Her only medication is the oral contraceptive pill.

Hb 10.3 g/dl, WBC 32 × 10^9/l, Platelets 430 × 10^9/l.

What explanations, based on the given data, can you offer to explain the patient's chest discomfort?

2. A 62 year old retired blacksmith presents with a 2 day history of tight chest pain and dyspnoea on exertion. The only abnormality on examination is a firm mobile node in the left axilla.

Urea 6.7 mmol/l, sodium 138 mmol/l, potassium 4.4 mmol/l, Bilirubin 23 μmol/l, ALT 31 U/l, Alk. Phos. 92 U/l, LDH 490 U/l, Total protein 71 g/l, Albumin 42 g/l.

(a) *What is the differential diagnosis?*

(b) *ECG and chest X–ray are normal — does this exclude any of your differential diagnosis?*

3. A 24 year old woman has presented with severe central chest and epigastric discomfort and her blood pressure is 200/125 mmHg. Another marked complaint is of breathlessness. Her peak expiratory flow rate is 90 litres/min. Forced expiratory volume in 1 second is 0.4 litres. Forced vital capacity is 3.6 litres.

(a) *What is the likely diagnosis?*

(b) *What confirmatory tests would you perform?*

4. A 62 year old businessman presents to his general practitioner with a 3 week history of dyspnoea and one week of palpitation. He is found to be in atrial fibrillation with left ventricular failure, and is treated with digoxin and frusemide. However his ventricular rate responds poorly to digoxin and he is referred for further assessment.

Plasma values: urea 22.2 mmol/l, sodium 128 mmol/l, potassium 3.4 mmol/l, bilirubin 16 μmol/l, alk. phos. 110 U/l, ALT 42 U/l.

(a) *What is the differential diagnosis?*

(b) *What further investigations are indicated?*

The following are normal ranges:
Plasma active renin concentration 9–50 μU/ml.
Plasma angiotensin II concentration 5–35 pg/ml.
Plasma aldosterone concentration less than 18 ng%.

5. A hypertensive 30 year old woman has presented with the following biochemical results:

Serum urea 3.6 mmol/l, sodium 146 mmol/l, potassium 2.4 mmol/l and bicarbonate 33 mol/l. Plasma renin, angiotensin II and aldosterone concentrations are 6 μU/ml, 5 pg/ml and 6 ng% respectively.

(a) *What is the provisional diagnosis based on the electrolyte picture?*

(b) *Do the hormone estimations confirm or exclude the diagnosis?*

(c) *What is the true diagnosis?*

(d) *How would you confirm the diagnosis?*

6. A 14 year old girl has a blood pressure, untreated, of 180/110 mmHg, while her plasma renin concentration is 290 μU/ml, plasma angiotensin II concentration 96 pg/ml and plasma aldosterone concentration is 40 ng %.

(a) *What is the differential diagnosis?*

(b) *Name two helpful tests in reaching the final diagnosis.*

7. What hypotensive drug treatment is likely to have been administered if the following plasma hormone concentrations are present?

(a) *Renin 90 μU/ml, angiotensin II 2 pg/ml, aldosterone 3 ng%.*

(b) *Renin 30 μU/ml, angiotensin II 18 pg/ml, aldosterone 40 ng%.*

8. A 23 year old housewife has just discovered she is seven weeks pregnant, but she presents to her general practitioner because of palpitation and lightheadedness. On referral to hospital she recalls a minor respiratory infection one week before the palpitation began. A 24 hour ambulatory ECG recording shows paroxysmal atrial tachycardia with block. A viral antibody screen yields the following titres:

Coxsackie B	1:8
C. Burneti	1:64
E.B. virus	1:16
Mycoplasma pneumoniae	1:8

(a) *What is the significance of these results?*

(b) *What form should your management take?*

9. The following data have been recorded before and after a diagnostic procedure in the catheter laboratory.

	Pressure (mmHg)	
	Before	**After**
RA	6	8
RV	44/8	56/10
PA	26/4	20/4
PA Wedge	16	—
LV	156/12	180/20
Aorta	134/92	106/74

(a) Which procedure has been employed?

(b) What is the diagnosis?

10. A 69 year old woman with a long history of ischaemic heart disease is admitted in pulmonary oedema which is treated with intravenous frusemide and 35% O_2 therapy. Next morning her chest is clearer but she looks cyanosed.

Plasma — urea 10.8 mmol/l, sodium 132 mmol/l, potassium 3.8 mmol/l.
Arterial blood gases pCO_2 16 kPa, pO_2 15 kPa, hydrogen ion 64 nmol/l, bicarbonate 36 mmol/l.

(a) What is the diagnosis?

(b) What is the treatment of choice?

11. The following results have been obtained in a 46 year old soldier whose blood pressure is 220/115 mmHg:

Haemoglobin 18.4 g/dl, haematocrit 54%, white cell count 9.2×10^9/l, platelets 180×10^9/l, serum urea 14 mmol/l.

(a) What is the differential diagnosis?

(b) What four tests would you find most helpful in reaching the diagnosis?

12. A treated hypertensive woman has presented to her general practitioner with tiredness. Her haemoglobin is 8.2 g/dl with normal white cell and platelet counts and absolute values. A reticulocyte count of 4% is noted. There is no evidence of blood loss.

(a) Which drug is most likely to have been used?

(b) Which single test will be most helpful in confirming your impression?

13. A 30 year old woman with odd behaviour has complained of a tender left knee joint. Her blood pressure is 260/150 mmHg while her haemoglobin is 5.6 g/dl with a reticulocyte count of 16%.

(a) What is the differential diagnosis?

(b) What further tests are indicated?

14. The following data have been recorded during cardiac catheterization in a 26 year old man:

Site	Pressure (mmHg)	O_2 saturation (%)
SVC	—	76
RA	8	77
RV	60/10	85
PA	58/16	83
PA Wedge	14	—
LV	122/22	91
Aorta	116/82	90

(a) *What is the diagnosis?*

(b) *What ECG abnormalities are likely in this patient?*

15. A 79 year old man has become progressively less mobile since the death of his wife 6 months before. On admission he is jaundiced, with a high JVP, hepatomegaly, bilateral pitting leg oedema, and a third heart sound.

Plasma results:- urea 7.4 mmol/l, sodium 134 mmol/l, potassium 2.5 mmol/l, bilirubin 56 μmol/l, Alk. phos. 170 U/l, ALT 92 U/l, AST 76 U/l, LDH 1043 U/l, Total protein 62 g/l, Albumin 28 g/l.

(a) *What is the differential diagnosis?*

(b) *Which invasive investigations, if any, are indicated?*

ANSWERS AND DISCUSSION

DATA

1. (a) Sternal ache due to leukaemic infiltration.
    (b) Leukaemoid reactions in the peripheral blood may be associated with S.L.E. (joint pain), infectious mononucleosis (again with joint discomfort, and characteristically presenting with sore throat), metastatic disease especially secondary to renal or bronchial carcinoma (sternal ache) or tuberculosis (sternal ache).
    (c) Severe infection of cardiac valves with associated angina — unlikely in view of presentation.
    (d) Premature coronary artery disease (oral contraceptive, and anaemia being contributory factors) in a patient with any of the conditions listed (a)–(c).

2. (a) i. Myocardial infarction.
        ii. Pulmonary enbolism (elevated bilirubin and LDH).
        iii. Ischaemic heart disease in a patient with early neoplastic infiltration of the liver (and axillary gland).
    (b) ECG may be normal in all the differentials, as may chest X–ray — if secondary deposits have not grown in lungs or mediastinum.

3. (a) Acute intermittent porphyria. The severe restrictive abnormality of respiratory function is secondary to a neuropathy affecting the phrenic and intercostal nerves. This patient could not even extinguish a match.
    (b) Ehrlich's aldehyde test is a useful sideroom test. Specific measures in urine of δ-aminolaevulinic acid, porphobilinogen, uroporphyrin and coproporphyrin are more accurate, and all should be elevated in the acute attack.

4. (a) The low urea effectively excludes diuretic excess as the cause for this patient's hyponatraemia. Inappropriate antidiuretic hormone secretion from a bronchial neoplasm with malignant infiltration of the heart precipitating atrial fibrillation is a likely explanation. That liver dysfunction could explain the biochemical abnormalities is belied by the moderate ALT level.
   (b) Plasma and urine osmolality; water load test; ADH assay; chest X–ray; ECG.
   Sputum cytology.
   Further biochemical tests of liver function, e.g. gamma GT.
   Serum thyroxine (a common cause of poor control with digoxin).

5. (a) Primary hyperaldosteronism — Conn's syndrome.
   (b) The hormone values do not confirm this impression, though they do not exclude it since secretion of aldosterone from a tumour may be episodic.
   (c) Either ingestion of exogenous mineralocorticoid such as liquorice or primary hyperaldosteronism with episodic secretion of hormone.
   (d) A careful dietary history. Four hourly blood samples for plasma aldosterone concentration to assess any diurnal change.

6. (a) i. Malignant phase hypertension. A blood pressure of 180/110 mmHg is very high for a 14 year old girl.
   ii. Renovascular hypertension.
   iii. Renin secreting tumour.
   (b) Renal arteriography.
   Renal vein sampling for plasma renin concentration.

7. (a) Converting enzyme inhibitor.
   (b) Spironolactone or amiloride.

8. (a) A single titre unless it is extremely high is difficult to interpret. This patient has probably experienced the usually mild respiratory infection of Q fever at some time in the past.

(b) i. A second sample for viral antibodies.
ii. Careful clinical and echocardiographic scrutiny of the patient's valves.
iii. Control of the arrhythmia if symptoms are troublesome — with beta blocker ± digoxin, avoiding medication in the first trimester if possible though neither agent is a recognised teratogen.

9. (a) Injection of inotrope, probably isoprenaline.
(b) The features are characteristic of hypertrophic cardiomyopathy with gradients across both aortic and pulmonary outflow tracts exacerbated by inotrope.

10. (a) Acute on chronic respiratory failure caused unwittingly by (for this patient) high concentrations of O_2, given reasonably during the presenting problem of pulmonary oedema. Arterial gases on air on admission would probably have alerted the clinician to the underlying complaint.
(b) Reduce inspired O_2 concentration.
Stimulate respiration with doxapram infusion (but note volume of infusate and the patient's recent pulmonary oedema).
Continue diuretics.

11. (a) The haematology results are indicative of secondary polycythaemia. The main differential diagnosis therefore rests between a primary respiratory problem, such as chronic obstructive airways disease causing polycythaemia in a patient with hypertensive renal damage, and primary renal disease such as polycystic kidneys or renal artery stenosis leading to renal impairment and polycythaemia and secondarily to hypertension.
(b) Respiratory function tests, chest X–ray and arterial blood gases would all be helpful in delineating an underlying respiratory problem. Intravenous urography would be most helpful as an initial step in identifying underlying renal disease.

12. (a) Alpha-methyldopa.
    (b) Coomb's test. Note that 15–20% of patients taking methyldopa develop a positive Coomb's test, often after 3 to 6 months of treatment, and more frequently when high doses of the drug are administered; however, only 5% of patients develop overt haemolytic anaemia, such as the patient described.

13. (a) i. Malignant phase hypertension with microangiopathic haemolytic anaemia (MAHA) and a bleeding tendency producing haemarthrosis. The unusual behaviour may be due to cerebral oedema.
    ii. Systemic lupus erythematosus producing both cerebral and joint symptoms as well as malignant phase hypertension with MAHA, or malignant phase hypertension and warm antibody type haemolytic anaemia, the latter being a further manifestation of SLE.
    (b) Blood film; platelet count; fibrinogen levels; fibrin degradation products. Antinuclear factor; DNA binding capacity; complement levels.

14. (a) Ventricular septal defect with mild pulmonary hypertension.
    (b) Right ventricular hypertrophy and strain.
    Right atrial hypertrophy.
    Left ventricular hypertrophy may also be present.
    Deep Q waves over V_5, V_6 are suggestive of V.S.D.

15. (a) i. Congestive cardiac failure with secondary hyperaldosteronism.
    ii. Dietary deficiencies leading to hypokalaemia and probable macrocytic anaemia as suggested by the disproportionately high LDH level and the deteriorating mobility (? myeloneuropathy). In view of the time course folate deficiency is likely. The anaemia will certainly exacerbate the cardiac failure.
    (b) Bone marrow aspiration.

PICTURES

Answers are on pages 219–220

QUESTIONS

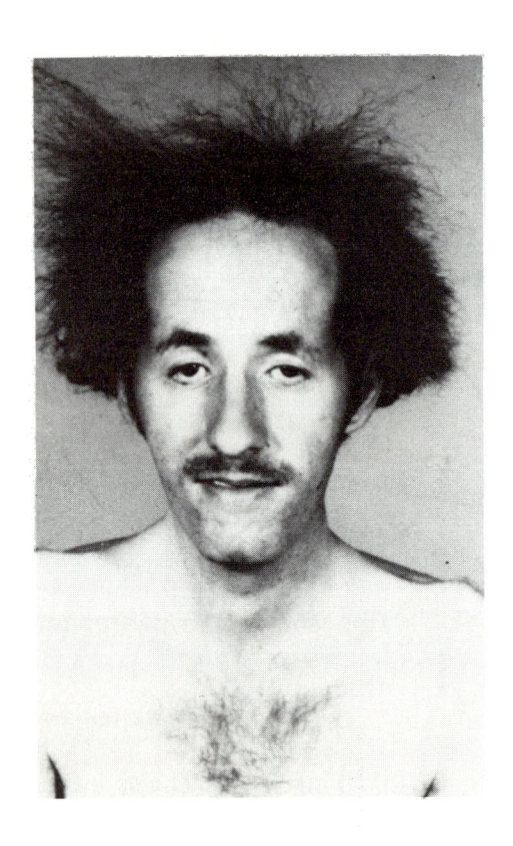

1. Figure 47
(a) *From which condition does this patient suffer?*
(b) *He has presented following an episode of collapse while crossing the road. What explanation(s) is/are likely?*
(c) *Are any relatives likely to be similarly affected, and if so, what mode of inheritance is involved?*

PICTURE QUIZ 217

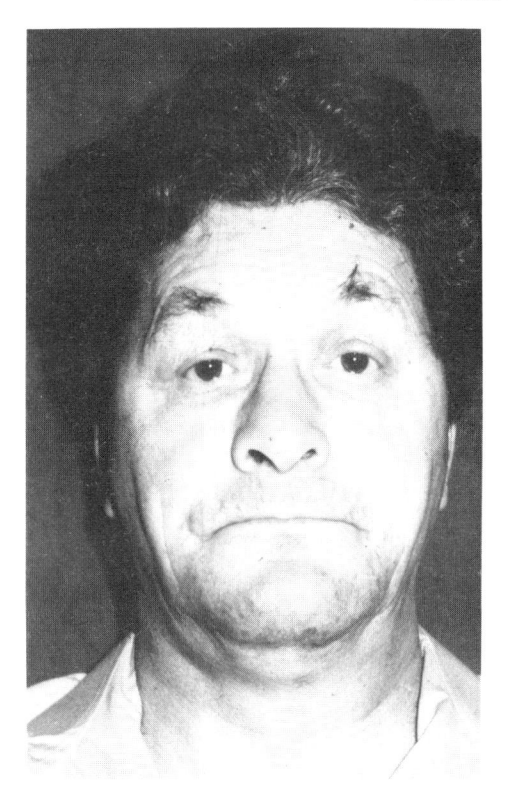

2. Figure 48
(a) What ECG abnormalities, if any, are likely in this patient?
(b) Hb 11.3 g/dl, MCV 102 fl, MCH 33 pg, MCHC 35 g/dl, urea 6.6 mmol/l, sodium 129 mmol/l, potassium 3.2 mmol/l. Are these (i) haematology, (ii) biochemistry results compatible with the clinical diagnosis, and if so, explain the basis of their compatibility?

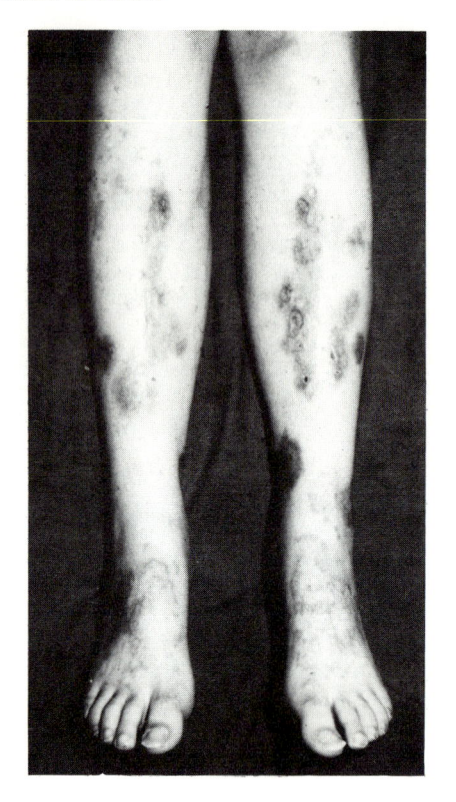

3. Figure 49

The patient whose legs are depicted in Figure 49 has been admitted with haematemesis and melaena thought to be due to salicylate ingestion. Blood pressure 100/60 mmHg in the right arm, lying. Pulse 70/min, regular. Hb. 9.8 g/dl with normal absolute values.

(a) *What does the clinical photograph show?*

(b) *Should this patient be transfused? Give reasons for your answer.*

ANSWERS AND DISCUSSION

PICTURES

1. (a) Dystrophia myotonica — characteristic expressionless face, with wasting of the facial muscles, and frontal balding.
    (b) Stokes-Adams attack caused by transient complete AV block.
    Paroxysmal atrial flutter/fibrillation.
    The sudden onset of the attack makes hypoglycaemia an unlikely explanation but patients with dystrophia myotonica often suffer from hyperinsulinism.
    (c) The trait is autosomal dominant with variable penetrance — the full syndrome includes testicular atrophy and infertility.
    Around 25% of patients are myotonic as the result of a new mutation.

2. (a) The patient with puffy coarse features and loss of the outer parts of his eyebrows is hypothyroid. Likely ECG abnormalities include sinus bradycardia, low voltage complexes, and any of the changes of ischaemic heart disease.
    (b) Both haematology and biochemistry results are compatible with hypothyroidism. The mild macrocytic anaemia may be due to the hypothyroidism itself, but one in eight patients with primary hypothyroidism suffer from pernicious anaemia also. A dilutional hyponatraemia is not uncommon in hypothyroidism.

3. (a) Necrobiosis lipoidica diabeticorum.
   (b) This patient is hypotensive and anaemic after a substantial gastrointestinal bleed. The bradycardia may well be due to autonomic dysfunction in this diabetic patient and may be masking the true extent of the blood loss.

ECHOCARDIOGRAMS

Answers are on page 224

QUESTIONS

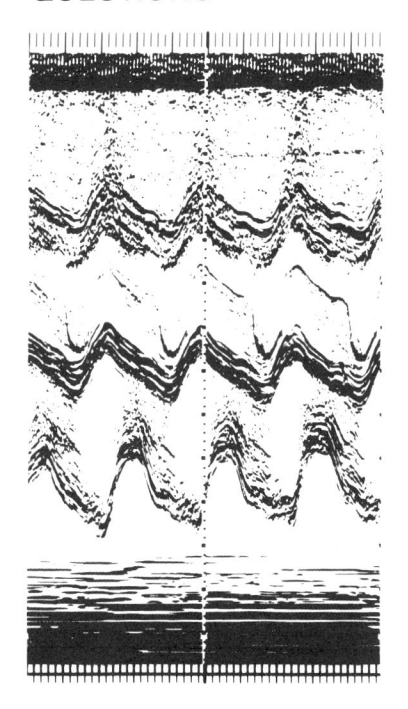

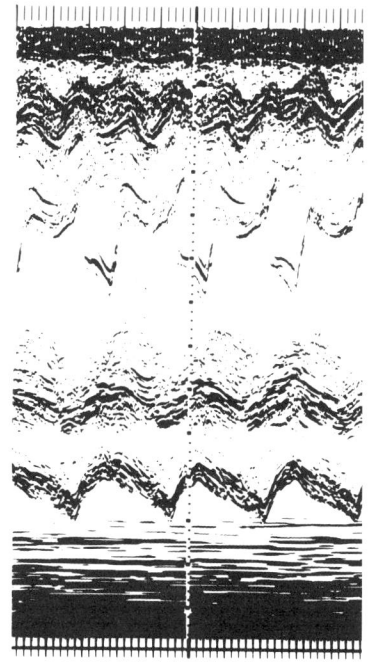

1. Figure 50
   Figure 50 shows the M-mode echocardiogram of a 64 year old woman with longstanding rheumatoid arthritis who has presented with pruritis and dyspnoea.

   (a) *What abnormalities are present?*
   (b) *What physical signs might you expect to detect?*

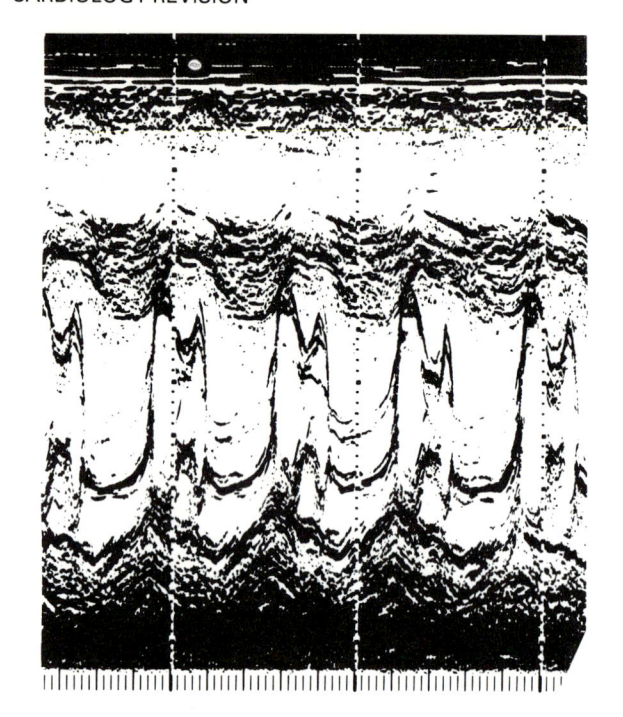

2. Figure 51
This echocardiogram has been recorded in a 29 year old man.

(a) What abnormalities are shown?

(b) Of which symptoms is the patient likely to complain?

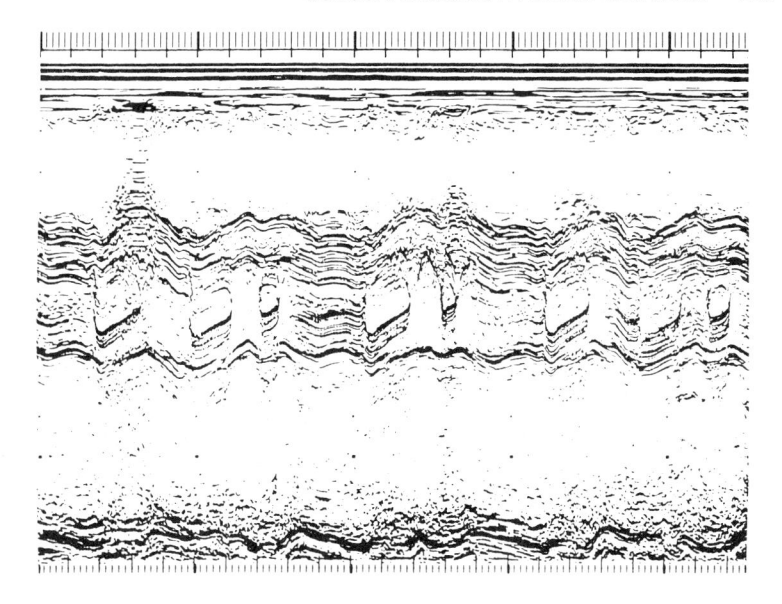

ECHOCARDIOGRAPHY INTERPRETATION 223

3. Figure 52
(a) *Describe this echocardiogram obtained from a 48 year old labourer.*

(b) *Apart from the chest X–ray and ECG, name the three investigations you think are most likely to help in the patient's management.*

ANSWERS AND DISCUSSION

ECHOCARDIOGRAMS

1. (a) A large anterior and small posterior pericardial effusion.
   (b) Characteristic findings in chronic effusion include tachycardia, hypotension, elevated JVP, hepatomegaly, peripheral oedema, pulsus paradoxus, quiet heart sounds, and often a pericardial rub.

2. (a) There is holosystolic prolapse of the posterior mitral valve leaflet producing a hammock shaped appearance. The left ventricle is hyperdynamic.
   (b) Most patients are asymptomatic. When symptoms occur palpitation, angina-like pain and stabbing pain at the apex may all occur.

3. (a) Multiple echoes arise from the anterior aortic wall and both the anterior but more markedly the posterior cusps of the aortic valve. The valve opens normally in systole (1.7 cm). The patient is in atrial fibrillation. The left atrium is slightly enlarged. The aortic appearance is characteristic of endocarditic vegetations.
   (b) Full blood count.
   ESR.
   Blood cultures.

3
LINKED CASES

PATIENT 1

Answers are on pages 230–231

HISTORY

A 75 year old retired gardener is admitted to the accident and emergency department after a fall in the street. Fortunately he has sustained no bony injury. He has no recall of this incident but admits to three blackouts over the previous year when out walking his dog. He denies any relationship of these episodes to sudden head or neck movement but admits that his dog is difficult to control and has often caused him to lose his balance. Over the previous 3 years he has noticed himself slowing up, and he becomes breathless on walking up hills. He is a widower, fiercely independent, and does all his own shopping and housework.

EXAMINATION

On examination his clothes are in poor repair, but he is clean shaven though thin and with clear evidence of weight loss. Memory and intellect normal. Ankle jerks absent bilaterally and plantars equivocal. Blood pressure 180/105 mmHg in the right arm lying. Pulse regular 76/min, good volume. Loud crowing ejection systolic murmur over the whole praecordium, maximal at apex, but conducted weakly to the right carotid artery, and more strongly to the left carotid.

QUESTIONS

1. Which of the following clinical deductions are true?

(a) *The findings are strongly suggestive of significant aortic stenosis.*

(b) *The neurological findings are consistent with a diagnosis of parasagittal meningioma complicated by epilepsy.*

(c) *A history of recent respiratory infection is irrelevant.*

(d) *Further investigation is mandatory.*

(e) *The absence of a definite relationship with head/neck movements excludes vertebrobasilar insufficiency as the cause of the lapses of consciousness.*

FURTHER INVESTIGATIONS

The patient consents to further investigation in the accident department. Cervical spine X–ray shows loss of disc space at C3/4, C4/5 and C5/6 levels with marked osteophytosis at C4/5. ECG normal. Plasma results — urea 8.2 mmol/l; Na 136 mmol/l; K 3.0 mmol/l; glucose 4.5 mmol/l.

QUESTIONS

2. Are the following conclusions justified?

(a) *A myocardial infarction has been excluded.*

(b) *The X–ray findings conclusively point to spondylosis as the underlying cause of the 'turns'.*

(c) *While on a cardiac monitor, pressure is applied to the carotid sinus with, after 10 seconds, sinus bradycardia, hypotension and dizziness — this implies that carotid sinus hypersensitivity is the likely cause of the 'turns'.*

(d) *Hypoglycaemia has satisfactorily been excluded as the cause of the 'turns'.*

(e) *Electrolyte results suggest that the patient has been taking diuretics.*

Because he is concerned about his dog the patient refuses to be admitted to hospital. He consents to outpatient investigation however, and a 24 hour ambulatory ECG recording, subsequently shows two episodes of atrial fibrillation with a ventricular rate of 100–120/minute lasting 30 seconds each. Unfortunately the patient has failed to note the times when he felt lightheaded during the period of the recording.

QUESTIONS

3. Does the registrar who subsequently reviews him at the outpatient department conclude correctly:

(a) *that digoxin 0.25 mg once daily is the treatment of choice*

(b) *that disopyramide is a suitable alternative if digoxin causes intolerable side effects*

(c) *that the patient may safely be discharged from the clinic, diagnosis paroxysmal atrial fibrillation*

(d) *that further investigation is warranted at this juncture*

(e) *that the results of an echocardiogram are unlikely to influence the patient's management?*

MANAGEMENT

The patient is commenced on digoxin 0.25 mg once daily but is readmitted before his next appointment complaining of dizziness and nausea. Blood pressure 170/90; pulse 45/min regular; no clinical or radiological evidence of left ventricular failure. ECG shows complete heart block.

QUESTIONS

4. Which of the following statements is/are true?

(a) *A temporary pacemaker should be inserted without delay.*

(b) *Further blood tests are not now important.*

(c) *A further 24 hour tape is indicated if permanent pacing is being contemplated.*

(d) *The findings are suggestive of vertebrobasilar insufficiency.*

(e) *Cardiac enzymes should be rechecked.*

The registrar on call decides to insert a temporary pacemaker and stop digoxin. 2 days later the patient feels much better, and is keen to have a permanent pacemaker implanted so that his turns can be stopped once and for all. He has returned to sinus rhythm, however, and a further 24 hour tape shows no abnormality.

QUESTIONS

5. Proper action now involves:

(a) *proceeding to implant a permanent pacemaker*

(b) *recording a further 24 hour tape before allowing the patient home*

(c) *a potassium supplemented diet*

(d) *a trial of a cervical collar*

(e) *reintroduction of digoxin at 0.125 mg o.d*

The decision is reached not to insert a permanent pacemaker. The temporary pacemaker is removed, but just as the patient is due to be discharged from the ward he suddenly collapses. The resident finds he has right sided hyperreflexia, with an extensor right plantar but flexor left plantar.

QUESTIONS

6. Which of the following statements is/are true?

(a) *The patient may have suffered an embolic stroke secondary to withdrawal of the temporary pacemaker.*

(b) A rapid return of the signs to normal within 12 hours shows that anticoagulation is warranted.

(c) The latest neurological event could not have been reasonably predicted on the basis of any of the previous history or examination.

(d) One paediatric aspirin tablet daily may be beneficial.

(e) It may be 'bolting the stable door' but a permanent pacemaker should now be implanted.

ANSWERS AND DISCUSSION

PATIENT 1

1. FALSE FALSE FALSE FALSE FALSE

The large pulse pressure makes significant aortic stenosis unlikely. Bilateral hyperreflexia at the ankles might suggest a parasagittal lesion. Cough syncope may be relevant in this patient. Further investigation is certainly desirable, but many old folk may wish to decline the offer of further interference. The patient's awareness of a relationship between head/neck movements and syncope is not always acute.

2. FALSE FALSE FALSE FALSE TRUE

ECG abnormalities may not develop for some hours after a myocardial infarction has occurred. Spondylosis is a very common finding in asymptomatic elderly people. Carotid sinus sensitivity is normal — and often the basis of a useful therapeutic gesture — but hypersensitivity will result in collapse after minor pressure such as that applied by a high collar. Many blood samples at a variety of times throughout the day and night may be necessary to exclude hypoglycaemia. The mild rise in urea and fall in potassium suggest diuretics may have been ingested.

3. FALSE   FALSE   FALSE   TRUE   FALSE

Digoxin may be an unnecessary (and potentially toxic) imposition if the arrhythmia is unrelated to symptoms. Disopyramide may cause postural hypotension and further confuse the situation. The diagnosis is not yet firm. If severe aortic stenosis is demonstrated surgical intervention may still be contemplated at this age. Repeat ambulatory monitoring is indicated.

4. FALSE   FALSE   TRUE   FALSE   TRUE

The patient is maintaining a satisfactory blood pressure, and since digoxin toxicity is likely withdrawal of that drug may be all that is required. Passage of a temporary pacing electrode in patients who are digoxin toxic may precipitate refractory arrhythmias. Alternative causes of heart block such as myocardial infarction should be excluded by cardiac enzyme estimation, and the serum digoxin level checked. There is still not enough evidence to warrant permanent pacing, and a further 24 hour tape recording should be made with the patient's pacemaker, if it has been inserted, set at 40/minute.

5. FALSE   TRUE   TRUE   TRUE   FALSE

While further evidence of arrhythmia sufficient to warrant permanent pacing is lacking, other therapeutic interventions are indicated — hypokalaemia should be corrected, and a trial of a cervical collar may abolish the attacks if indeed cervical spondylosis is the correct aetiology.

6. TRUE   FALSE   FALSE   TRUE   FALSE

Thrombus may form on the left ventricular side of the septum opposite the site at which the temporary electrode has been positioned in the right ventricle. The likely explanation is an embolus from the patient's left carotid artery — remember the inequality in the systolic bruits over the carotid vessels — and treatment with aspirin and dipyridamole indicated rather than anticoagulation. There is still no evidence that the patient should receive a permanent pacemaker.

PATIENT 2

Answers are on pages 237–238

HISTORY

An obese 66 year old non-insulin dependent diabetic woman is admitted to the coronary care unit with a 4 hour history of severe retrosternal heaviness radiating to the jaw, with nausea, sweating and worsening dyspnoea. She has never experienced similar complaints before, but in the past has undergone femoral herniorrhaphy, vaginal hysterectomy, and ligation of varicose veins, and has suffered from a hiatus hernia for 10 years. Medication on admission — chlorpropamide 250 mg daily, antacid. Social history — Jehovah's witness, non-smoker, non-drinker; her husband, a retired teacher, is in good health.

EXAMINATION

On examination she is obese. Arcus corneae. Pinpoint pupils bilaterally. Tendon reflexes symmetrical. Plantars flexor. Blood pressure 110/60 mmHg in the right arm, lying. Pulse 110/min regular. Third heart sound present. No murmurs. Widespread fine crepitations in both lungs.

ECG: sinus tachycardia, evolving anterior myocardial infarction.

Chest X–ray: alveolar oedema.

QUESTIONS

1. Which of the following statements regarding the emergency treatment of this patient is/are true?

(a) *Intravenous isosorbide infusion is the initial treatment of choice.*

(b) *Intravenous frusemide provides symptomatic relief before any diuresis occurs.*

(c) *Opiate should be withheld unless the patient experiences chest pain.*

(d) *Because of the tachycardia parenteral beta blockade is indicated.*

(e) *Digoxin 0.5 mg intravenously is indicated to control tachycardia and relieve cardiac failure.*

FURTHER MANAGEMENT

Over the next 6 hours the patient experiences a satisfactory diuresis with relief of dyspnoea after frusemide 50 mg intravenously. She also receives cyclimorph 5 mg i.v., but in view of her history of hiatus hernia is not anticoagulated. She then experiences two short runs of ventricular tachycardia (12 and 15 beats) associated with lightheadedness and is given two boluses of lignocaine 100 mg i.v. while an infusion of lignocaine is set up. Following a further breakthrough run of ventricular tachycardia 30 minutes later she receives a further bolus of lignocaine 100 mg i.v.

QUESTIONS

2. Regarding her further management:

(a) *the treatment of choice may be parenteral potassium*

(b) *28% or 35% oxygen must be administered*

(c) *agitation is likely to be due to hypoglycaemia*

(d) *naloxone is unlikely to prevent further arrhythmia*

(e) *oral loading doses of amiodarone are indicated at this juncture.*

Following modification of her antiarrhythmic regimen no further tachycardia occurs. However the third heart sound persists, and systolic pressure runs at between 110 and 120 mmHg, but urine output is well maintained. After 48 hours have elapsed the patient is transferred to the general ward. Next day she is noted to have a warm red tender swollen right calf, pyrexia (38.3°C), leucocytosis (12.4 × 10^9/l) and an elevated ESR (65 mm in one hour). Before anticoagulant can be commenced she becomes acutely unwell and is found to have right sided hyperreflexia and dysphasia.

QUESTIONS

3. Which of the following statements is/are true?

(a) *Paradoxical embolism from the deep calf veins is the likely explanation.*

(b) *A paradoxical impulse over the praecardium is unlikely to be important.*

(c) *Pulsus paradoxus will probably be present.*

(d) *If the neurological signs resolve within 6 hours, hypoglycaemia is the likely cause.*

(e) *Arteritis is a likely explanation for all of the cardiac and neurological problems.*

The patient is anticoagulated initially with heparin and then warfarin. The weakness improves but the dysphasia remains distressing. After 20 mg + 5 mg warfarin on successive days the prothrombin time ratio (PTR) the following morning is 1.1:1. A further 10 mg warfarin is administered but the PTR next morning is 1.3:1. After a further 5 mg warfarin the PTR remains at 1.3:1. After a further 5 mg the PTR is 10:1.

QUESTIONS

4. Likely cause(s) for these unusual results are:

(a) *hepatic congestion*

(b) *concurrent paracetamol for headache*

(c) *another patient of the same surname in the ward*

(d) *laboratory error*

(e) *constipation.*

To your dismay the patient develops melaena and her haemoglobin drops to 8.8 g/dl (13.2 g/dl on admission). Blood pressure is 120/70 mmHg and pulse 100/min regular.

QUESTIONS

5. The optimum treatment is:

(a) *cautious transfusion of packed cells*

(b) *transfusion of whole blood plus diuretics*

(c) *oral iron and parenteral vitamin K*

(d) *observation only with recheck of haemoglobin later that day*

(e) *parenteral vitamin K in addition to transfusion of packed cells.*

Eventually the patient is discharged home on chlorpropamide, frusemide, mexiletine and slow-release potassium. She receives outpatient physiotherapy and is reviewed regularly at medical outpatients. However the patient is troubled by dyspnoea often on exertion but sometimes at rest also. Her ECG at outpatient review 3 months after the myocardial infarction is shown in figure 53.

236 CARDIOLOGY REVISION

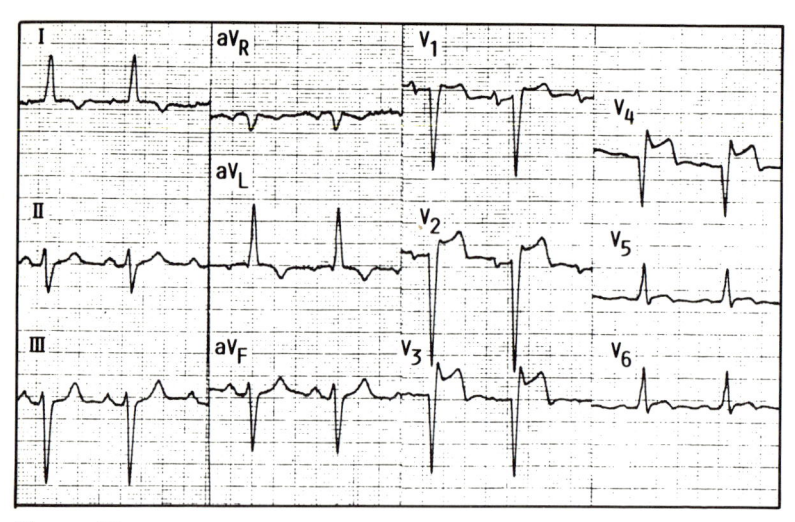

Figure 53

QUESTIONS

6. In view of the foregoing information:

(a) digoxin is now clearly the treatment of choice

(b) a 24 hour ambulatory ECG recording is an unnecessary expense

(c) domiciliary oxygen therapy is indicated

(d) longterm beta-blocker prophylaxis is contraindicated

(e) mexiletine ought to have been withdrawn 4 weeks after the infarct.

ANSWERS AND DISCUSSION

PATIENT 2

1. FALSE   TRUE   FALSE   FALSE   FALSE

In the initial treatment of pulmonary oedema morphine (because of central and vasodilator effects) and frusemide (because of pulmonary vasodilator and diuretic effects) with high flow oxygen are most helpful. Isosorbide may indeed be helpful by reducing preload but is not the initial treatment of choice. Beta blockade will have further cardiac depressant effects and is undesirable — the tachycardia is appropriate given the clinical circumstances. Digoxin is not very helpful while the patient is in sinus rhythm.

2. TRUE   FALSE   FALSE   TRUE   FALSE

Hypokalaemia prevents effective action of lignocaine. High flow oxygen is indicated in the absence of chronic respiratory disease. In this acute illness the patient is likely to be hyperglycaemic and may require a sliding scale insulin regimen for a few days. Amiodarone is not indicated but a change to mexiletine may be helpful.

3. FALSE   FALSE   FALSE   FALSE   FALSE

The likely explanation is embolism of mural thrombus, and this is all the more likely if a ventricular aneurysm (paradoxical pulsation) is developing.

4. FALSE   FALSE   FALSE   FALSE   TRUE

Marked intestinal stasis in this patient who is currently bedbound may lead to interference with absorption of warfarin. The 'rebound' anticoagulation in this case followed administration of laxatives.

5. FALSE FALSE TRUE FALSE FALSE

Whatever the medical opinion, nontransfusion is the optimum treatment allowed by this patient since she is a Jehovah's witness. Control of coagulation should be sought with vitamin K and oral iron.

6. FALSE FALSE FALSE TRUE FALSE

The ECG shows persistent anterior ST segment elevation suggesting that a left ventricular aneurysm is present.

Digoxin is not indicated since it is not known if an arrhythmia which is digitalis-responsive is present. A 24 hour recording is a very useful test, but the mechanical effect of the aneurysm without associated tachyarrhythmia may be the only aetiological factor. Given the cardiac failure, beta-blockade is contraindicated, but since ventricular arrhythmias are common in this condition withdrawal of mexiletine must be weighed up very carefully.

PATIENT 3

Answers are on pages 243–245

HISTORY

A 73 year old retired lawyer presents with a 2 month history of malaise, dyspnoea at night and on exertion, painful bilateral ankle swelling of increasing magnitude, and nausea. He gives no history of past medical illnesses, but has been depresssed since the death of his wife 6 months previously. He denies abuse of alcohol and has never smoked. On systems enquiry he confesses to symptoms of prostatism, constipation and insomnia. He denies ingestion of any medication.

EXAMINATION

Examination shows him to have icteric sclerae and scratch marks on arms and abdomen. He wears his wife's watch on his left wrist. Central cyanosis. JVP + 15 cm. Pitting oedema of ankles, thighs and abdominal wall. Blood pressure 110/80 mmHg in left arm, lying. Pulse 94/minute, irregular. Apex beat in sixth intercostal space in midaxillary line. Heart sounds faint, but third sound present. Grade 2/6 mid-systolic murmur at base poorly conducted. Abdomen — mild ascites; liver edge 8 cm below costal margin; spleen not felt. Respiratory — widespread coarse crepitations.

QUESTIONS

1. The physical findings are compatible with a diagnosis of

(a) alcoholic liver disease

(b) paracetamol overdosage

(c) aortic stenosis

(d) congestive cardiac failure

(e) chronic pulmonary thromboembolism.

FURTHER INVESTIGATIONS

ECG shows sinus rhythm with supraventricular and ventricular ectopics, low voltage complexes, left axis deviation and widespread repolarization abnormalities.

QUESTIONS

2. Which of the following statements is/are true?

(a) The ECG is compatible with alcoholic cardiomyopathy.

(b) Left axis deviation implies left anterior hemiblock in this patient.

(c) A beat to beat alteration in the height of the QRS complexes is additional evidence of congestive cardiac failure.

(d) The ECG findings are characteristic of end stage aortic stenosis.

(e) The absence of right heart strain excludes a diagnosis of pulmonary emboli.

Chest X–ray confirms the clinical impression of cardiomegaly and pulmonary oedema with, in addition, a small pleural effusion at the right base. The biochemical picture obtained from plasma: urea 14.2 mmol/l, sodium 130 mmol/l, potassium 3.0 mmol/l, bicarbonate 28 mmol/l, bilirubin 67 μmol/l, alkaline phosphatase 160 U/l, ALT 90 U/l, AST 82 U/l, LDH 543 U/l, protein 62 g/l, albumin 29 g/l, thyroxine 56 nmol/l.

QUESTIONS

3. Which of the following statements is/are true?

(a) An infusion of plasma will help to clear the oedema.

(b) If fasting triglycerides are 10.6 mmol/l, alcohol excess will be the likely diagnosis.

(c) Myocardial infarction is excluded by the biochemical results.

(d) Hypoalbuminaemia is a sensitive index of subacute or chronic liver disease.

(e) The biochemical picture is all explicable in terms of hypothyroidism.

4. Given the clinical and biochemical findings which of the following are likely to be elevated?

(a) Plasma volume.

(b) Total exchangeable sodium.

(c) Total exchangeable potassium.

(d) Plasma renin concentration.

(e) Extracellular fluid volume.

5. In view of the findings which further investigations are indicated?

(a) Two-dimensional echocardiography.

(b) Exercise tolerance test.

(c) Coronary angiography.

(d) Pulmonary function tests.

(e) Liver biopsy.

MANAGEMENT

The patient is treated aggressively with frusemide 80 mg b.d. orally and spironolactone 100 mg b.d. orally. Despite this over the next 2 days his weight increases by a further 2 kg.

QUESTIONS

6. Likely explanations for the weight gain are
(a) *non-compliance*
(b) *spironolactone does not begin to work properly for 48 hours*
(c) *malabsorption*
(d) *deterioration in renal function*
(e) *severe secondary hyperaldosteronism.*

7. Useful manoeuvres given the failure of diuretics include:
(a) *confinement to bed*
(b) *fluid restriction*
(c) *salt restriction*
(d) *parenteral diuretics*
(e) *oral sodium bicarbonate.*

Next evening the resident is called to see the patient who is vomiting and complaining of palpitation — an ECG confirms that the patient is now in atrial fibrillation. The resident opts to digitalize the patient with 0.5 mg digoxin intravenously in 250 ml normal saline.

8. How much sodium does this infusion contain?
(a) *10 mmol.*
(b) *15 mmol.*
(c) *20 mmol.*

(d) *40 mmol.*

(e) *80 mmol.*

2 days later the patient reverts to sinus rhythm with ventricular ectopics. These ectopics occur 10 times/minute and the question of whether they should be suppressed pharmacologically is raised.

9. Which of the following statements is/are true?

(a) *Radionudide ventriculography will provide an answer as to the effect of these ectopics on cardiac output.*

(b) *Ectopics occurring with this frequency are unlikely to influence cardiac output.*

(c) *A 24 hour ECG recording will be a helpful investigation.*

(d) *Echocardiography is a useful quantitative test in these circumstances.*

(e) *If treatment is contemplated and in view of the patient's previous supraventricular ectopics, disopyramide is the treatment of choice.*

ANSWERS AND DISCUSSION

PATIENT 3

1. FALSE   FALSE   TRUE   TRUE   FALSE

Alcoholic liver disease does not explain the left heart findings. The physical signs indicate a chronic disorder with oedema and ascites, and not acute paracetamol overdosage. Aortic stenosis may cause left and rarely predominantly right heart failure. The description is characteristic of congestive cardiac failure, but thromboembolism does not account for the left ventricular failure.

2. TRUE TRUE TRUE FALSE FALSE

In a normotensive patient left axis deviation implies left anterior hemiblock. Electrical alternans is typical of severe myocardial dysfunction. Severe aortic stenosis is usually associated with marked left ventricular hypertrophy. Pulmonary emboli often occur without associated ECG abnormality.

3. FALSE TRUE FALSE TRUE FALSE

Plasma will produce more marked pulmonary oedema. Hypertriglyceridaemia is a characteristic finding of alcoholic fatty hepatitis. Myocardial infarction and right heart failure may coexist. Hypoalbuminaemia often implies chronic liver disease. Hypothyroidism may produce LDH elevation but not such generalized and marked liver dysfunction — a thyroxine level of 56 nmol/l is probably within normal limits for a patient of this age.

4. TRUE TRUE FALSE TRUE TRUE

Plasma volume may be marginally increased, and more so when the patient becomes supine at night. Although hyponatraemia is common sodium retention as far as the whole body is concerned may occur. Partly because of secondary hyperaldosteronism, with high renin levels also, exchangeable potassium is not usually increased. Extracellular fluid increases are manifested as ascites and peripheral oedema.

5. TRUE FALSE FALSE FALSE FALSE

None of the tests (b)–(e) are indicated, either because of the patient's age or because they are premature in a patient with a history very suggestive of congestive cardiac failure (CCF) in whom diuretic therapy may be successful. However CCF is not an adequate diagnosis, and its cause must be sought — to this end echocardiography may be useful and is noninvasive.

6. FALSE FALSE TRUE FALSE FALSE

The likely explanation is that the peripheral oedema is also affecting the patient's gut wall and preventing normal absorption of medication. It is a common fallacy that spironolactone does not work for several days — it works within hours, though the potassium sparing effects may not be reflected in plasma potassium levels for several days.

7. TRUE TRUE TRUE TRUE FALSE

Any measures designed to produce negative salt and water balance will be helpful. Confinement to bed often improves renal perfusion, and decreases the demands on the heart. The most useful measure is administration of diuretics parenterally — multiplication of medications designed to reduce preload and afterload cannot work if they are not absorbed through the intestinal mucosa either.

8. FALSE FALSE FALSE TRUE FALSE

The volume of the infusate is unnecessarily large, but it emphasizes the importance of appreciating the amount of sodium present in one litre of normal saline, i.e. 150 mmol.

9. FALSE FALSE TRUE FALSE FALSE

Frequent ectopics compromise interpretation of ejection fraction results obtained at radionuclide ventriculography. The frequency of the ectopics may be assessed by 24 hour taping, but it is likely that at the frequency noted cardiac output will be reduced. In these circumstances echocardiography does not provide helpful quantitative information. In view of the anticholinergic effects of disopyramide this drug is best avoided in a patient with prostatism.

PATIENT 4

Answers are on pages 250–252

HISTORY

A 45 year old baker is referred to the medical outpatient clinic with a 6 month history of tiredness. He has, however, no specific complaints on systems enquiry other than that he has been unable to undertake strenuous activity in his capacity as coach to a boys' football team without feeling exhausted. He is a non-smoker, denies alcohol abuse, is married but has no children and has worked on the night shift for 20 years. His only past history is of appendicectomy 15 years before.

QUESTIONS

1. Which of the following statements is/are true?

(a) The history is compatible with a diagnosis of adult coeliac disease.

(b) An 8 a.m. plasma cortisol level of 180 nmol/l is diagnostic of Addison's disease.

(c) Narcolepsy often presents in this way.

(d) In view of his occupation byssinosis is a possible explanation for his presentation.

(e) The presentation is characteristic of severe hypertension.

EXAMINATION

Blood pressure 110/80 mmHg in the right arm, lying. Pulse: sinus rhythm, 80/minute, small volume. Apex beat in fifth interspace 3 cm outside the midclavicular line. S_1 soft, S_2 single and quiet. Grade 2/6 ejection systolic murmur at apex, with systolic bruits in both carotid arteries.

Respiratory examination normal.

QUESTIONS

2. Which of the following statements is/are true?

(a) *The intensity of the murmur is a poor guide to the severity of the stenosis.*

(b) *Squatting will decrease and the Valsalva manoeuvre increase the intensity of the murmur.*

(c) *The absence of an ejection click implies calcification of the valve.*

(d) *Longer murmurs imply more severe stenosis.*

(e) *The mild symptoms imply a mild stenosis.*

FURTHER INVESTIGATIONS

At cardiac catheterization the following pressures are obtained (mmHg) — right atrium 6, right ventricle 34/6, main pulmonary artery 30/10, pulmonary artery wedge 18, left ventricle 190/20, ascending aorta 110/70.

QUESTIONS

3. Which of the following statements is/are true?

(a) *The laboratory data imply the stenosis is mild to moderate.*

(b) *Absence of left ventricular hypertrophy on the ECG suggests there is no significant stenosis.*

(c) *Aortic stenosis may be the result of a congenitally malformed tricuspid valve.*

(d) *Ventricular filling in aortic stenosis is impaired by increased muscle stiffness.*

(e) *Patients with aortic stenosis may present with right ventricular failure before developing left ventricular failure clinically.*

MANAGEMENT

The patient comes to aortic valve surgery and his aortic valve is replaced with a Bjork-Shiley prosthesis.

QUESTIONS

4. Which of the following statements regarding cardiac surgery are true?

(a) *During bypass surgery asystole may be induced by infusing cardioplegic solution at 4°C directly into the coronary ostia.*

(b) *Ultrastructural changes almost invariably occur in the cooled arrested heart.*

(c) *Cardioplegic solution contains high concentrations of potassium.*

(d) *Propranolol has adverse effects during cardioplegia.*

(e) *Varicose veins are unsuitable for grafting in coronary artery surgery.*

5. Which of the following statements regarding anticoagulation after cardiac surgery is/are true?

(a) *Anticoagulation is not indicated after coronary artery surgery.*

(b) *Patients receiving valve xenografts need not be anticoagulated.*

(c) *Concurrent atrial fibrillation does not increase the incidence of embolization in patients with xenografts.*

(d) *If a patient with a Starr-Edwards prosthesis becomes pregnant anticoagulation with warfarin should be continued through delivery.*

(e) *Anticoagulants effectively abolish embolic phenomena.*

8 months after surgery the patient is referred urgently from a peripheral hospital where he has been admitted cold, clammy, hypotensive (100/60), anuric and dyspnoeic after a 48 hour period of malaise and mild chest discomfort. His ECG shows T inversion in V_3–V_8.

QUESTIONS

6. Which of the following statements is/are true?

(a) *Previously undiagnosed coronary artery disease is a likely explanation.*

(b) *Obstruction of the prosthesis may be excluded by echocardiography.*

(c) *Dopamine infusion is an appropriate treatment.*

(d) *The patient should be treated with antibiotics as soon as blood cultures have been taken.*

(e) *Rectal examination may be helpful.*

ANSWERS AND DISCUSSION

PATIENT 3

1. TRUE   FALSE   FALSE   FALSE   FALSE

The characteristic features of adult coeliac disease at presentation nowadays are often nonspecific, or the result of anaemia, and severe gastrointestinal complaints less common. Since the patient has been on the night shift for 20 years an 8 a.m. cortisol may be his 'night time' value and a 4 p.m. value may be high. Narcolepsy presents at a younger age with frequent episodes of dropping off to sleep. Extrinsic allergic alveolitis may be an occupational hazard in bakers, but byssinosis is linked with cotton and hemp industries and does not have this presentation. Severe hypertension, unless malignant phase optic fundal changes and headache occur, is usually asymptomatic.

2. TRUE   FALSE   TRUE   TRUE   FALSE

The intensity of the systolic murmur and the severity of the symptoms are inaccurate guides to the severity of the stenosis. More severe stenoses produce longer murmurs which peak later in systole. Squatting increases the gradient and the intensity of the murmurs, while the Valsalva manoeuvre decreases the intensity of the murmur. Ejection clicks imply mobility of the cusps, a feature which disappears with calcification.

3. FALSE   TRUE   TRUE   TRUE   TRUE

With a peak systolic gradient of 80 mmHg the valve orifice is critically reduced to less than a fifth of its normal area and the stenosis is severe. Left ventricular hypertrophy is usually marked in significant stenosis unless the onset of the stenosis has been very rapid. Congenitally malformed unicuspid, bicuspid or tricuspid valves may all lead to stenosis. The hypertrophied left ventricular muscle produces a stiffness which hinders ventricular filling in diastole. If septal hypertrophy is marked this may impinge on the right ventricle and cause right heart failure — the so-called Bernheim effect.

4. TRUE   TRUE   TRUE   FALSE   TRUE

Cardioplegic solution containing high potassium concentrations is usually infused into the aortic root, but if aortic regurgitation is present direct infusion of 200–1000 ml directly into the coronary vessels may be necessary. Despite the protection afforded by cold cardioplegia ultrastructural damage invariably occurs, but propranolol has been found to have some protective effects.

In coronary artery bypass graft surgery varicose veins are unsuitable for grafting and sufferers may require arm veins to be used as grafts.

5. FALSE   FALSE   FALSE   FALSE   FALSE

After coronary endarterectomy prolonged anticoagulation is indicated. Most thromboembolic episodes in patients with mitral xenografts occur in the first 3 months after surgery, after which anticoagulants may be discontinued, unless a further thrombogenic factor such as left atrial enlargement or continuing atrial fibrillation exist. It must be appreciated that even with anticoagulation in patients with prosthetic valves, thromboembolism occurs in around 5% of patients per year. Pregnant patients should have heparin substituted for warfarin near term, and the heparin should be discontinued for the few days either side of elective delivery; ideally xenografts should be implanted in women of child-bearing age.

6. FALSE   TRUE   TRUE   FALSE   TRUE

The patient's coronary arteries will have been scrutinized prior to valve surgery (and grafted as necessary during a combined procedure). Echocardiography is very helpful in demonstrating normal prosthetic function. Inotropic support is clearly needed in this patient, but evidence of endocarditis will have been sought during echocardiography and without clear evidence of infection being present antibiotic therapy may be counterproductive at this stage. Faecal occult blood in stool or overt melaena on the glove may bring to light unexpected gastrointestinal blood loss, to which anticoagulant therapy may have contributed.

FURTHER READING

Birkenhager W H, Reid J L (eds) 1983 Handbook of hypertension. Elsevier/North Holland, Amsterdam

Braunwald E 1980 Heart disease — a textbook of cardiovascular medicine. W B Saunders, Philadelphia

Feigenbaum H 1982 Echocardiography, 3rd edn. Lea & Febiger, Philadelphia

Julian D G, Pentecost B 1981–1983 Medical international new series. Medical Education, Oxford, nos 17–20, pp 807–924

Opie L H 1980 Drugs and the heart, Lancet

Schamroth L 1982 An introduction to electro-cardiography, 3rd edn. Blackwell Scientific, Oxford

INDEX

Italics indicate a reference in the Interpretation section

Addison's disease, 111, 247
Alcohol, 4
Alcohol withdrawal, 159
Aldosterone, *208, 209, 213*
Amyloidosis, 111
Anatomy, cardiac, 38
Aneurysm, left ventricular, *169, 180, 237*
Angiotensin II, *208, 209, 213*
Aorta, ascending, *174, 182*
Aortic regurgitation, 20
Aortic stenosis, 37, 38, *248, 249*
Arrest, cardiac, 42
Arrhythmia, drug treatment, 98, 99
Arteriosclerosis obliterans, 158
Ascites, 240
Atherosclerosis, 81
Atrial fibrillation, 121, *183, 202*
Atrial septal defect, 134
A-V block, 103, 104, *196, 205,* 228
A-V dissociation, *193, 197, 203, 205*

Berry aneurysm, *181*
Beta-blockers, 48, 49, 104
'Blackouts', 226–232
Bornholm disease, 4, 5
Bradycardia, sinus, 43
Bronchiectasis, 111
Bruit, abdominal, 13
Bundle branch block, left, 70
Bundle branch block, right, *185, 201*
Byssinosis, 247

Calcium antagonists, 122, 123
Cardiac catheter data, *209, 211, 214, 215*
Cardiomegaly, *177, 178, 183*
Cardiomyopathy, 5
Cardiomyopathy, alcoholic, 115
Cardiomyopathy, drug related, 98
Cardiomyopathy, hypertrophic, 117, *209, 214*

Carotid sinus hypersensitivity, 227
Cerebral haemorrhage, 145
Cervical spondylosis, 227
Chagas disease, 123
Claudication, calf, 152
Coarctation of the aorta, *172, 181*
Coeliac disease, 247
Congenital heart disease, 134
Congestive cardiac failure, 38, 39, 104, 242
Converting enzyme inhibitor, 62, 75, 78
Coronary angiography, 140
Coronary artery disease — epidemiology, 81
Creatinine clearance, 93
Cushing's syndrome, 48

Debrisoquine, 48
Depression, 71
Dextrocardia, *184, 201*
Diabetes mellitus, 91, 123, 233
Diabetic ketoacidosis, 94
Digoxin, 65, 228
Dissection of the aorta, 21
Diuretics, 243
Dystrophia myotonica, *216, 219*

Ebstein's anomaly, 65
Electrocardiogram, low voltage, 139
Embolism, paradoxical, 135
Embolism, pulmonary, 98, *191, 203*
Exercise tolerance test, 64, 65, *186, 190, 192, 200, 202, 203, 206*
External cardiac massage, 70

Fibromuscular hyperplasia, *170, 180*
Folate deficiency, *211, 215*
Frank-Starling curve, 43
Frostbite, 158

Hydrallazine, 48

Hyperaldosteronism, primary, 31, 32, *213*
Hyperaldosteronism, secondary, 92
Hyperlipidaemia, 81
Hypertension, primary pulmonary, 70
Hypertension, systemic, 13, 14
  drug treatment, 49, 60, 92, 146
  investigation, 16, 49
  ischaemic heart disease in, 123
  malignant phase, 58, 59, 93
  pregnancy, 30, 31
  secondary, 109
  symptoms, 93
Hyperthyroidism, 141
Hypertrophy, left ventricular, 15, *192, 196, 203, 204*
Hypertrophy, right atrial, *195, 204*
Hypokalaemia, 91
Hyponatraemia, *208, 213*
Hyponatraemic hypertensive syndrome, 93
Hypotension, postural, 109, 110
Hypothermia, *189, 203*
Hypothyroidism, 37, 68, *217, 219*

Idioventricular rhythm, *187, 202*
Intravenous urography, 60
Ischaemia, renal, 77

Kidney, unilateral small, 129
Kyphoscoliosis, *167, 179*

Leukaemia, *212*
Leukaemoid reactions, *212*

Marfan's syndrome, 20
Methyldopa, 48, 110, *210, 215*
Mitral stenosis, 135
Mitral valve disease, *164, 179*
Mitral valve prolapse, 20, *222, 224*
Mitral valve prosthesis, *175, 182*
Morphine, 71
Murmur, mid-diastolic, 135
Myocardial infarction, 25, 26
  acute, 70, 86
  causes, 44
  convalescence, 43
  inferior, *190, 203*
  licences and, 28
  right ventricular, 105
  subendocardial, 71
  true posterior, *197, 205*
Myocarditis, 5
Myxoma, cardiac, 116

Narcolepsy, 247
Necrobiosis lipoidica diabeticorum, *218, 220*
Nephrectomy, unilateral, 129
Nitrates, 104
Node, sinoatrial, 26

Oral contraceptives, 31, 58

Pacemaker
  atrial, *185, 190, 201, 203*
  A-V sequential, *166, 179*
  temporary, 55, 65, 229, 230
  VAT, *191, 203*
  ventricular, 140, *187, 188, 189, 200, 202, 206*
Papillary muscle rupture, 88
Papilloedema, 146
Pericardial effusion, *221, 224*
Pericarditis, 151
Pericardiocentesis, 151
Petit mal epilepsy, *194, 204*
Phaeochromocytoma, 50, 145, 146, 147
Polycystic kidneys, *168, 180*
Polycythaemia, secondary, *210, 214*
Porphyria, 93, *212*
Prazosin, 48, 129
Pregnancy, 82
Prosthetic valves, 53, 54
Pseudophaeochromocytoma, 147
Pulmonary oedema, 43, 70, *173, 181*, 234
Pulmonary stenosis, 159
Pyrophosphate scan, 139

QT interval, prolonged, 122

Raynaud's phenomenon, 157
Renal artery stenosis, 59, 60, 76, *165, 176, 179, 182*
Renal failure, 75, 76
Renin, *208, 209, 213*
Respiratory failure, *210, 214*
Rheumatic fever, 115

S_2, 140
S_3, 4
Saline infusion, 243
Shoulder-hand syndrome, 27
Sick sinus syndrome, 157
Smoking, cigarette, 92
Spasm, coronary artery, 66, 87
Spironolactone, 32
Subacute bacterial endocarditis, 9

Subarachnoid haemorrhage, 71
Superior vena cava, left persisting, *171, 180*
Surgery, cardiac, 87, 249, 250
Suxamethonium, 100
Sympathomimetic drugs, 99
Systemic lupus erythematosus, *210, 215*

Tachycardia
　atrial, *192, 203*
　broad complex, *194, 204*
　ventricular, 234
Tamponade, acute cardiac, 103
Tape, 24-hour ambulatory ECG, 228
Theophylline toxicity, 141
Thiazides, 109
Thrombosis, deep venous, 152

Trauma, chest, 151
Tuberculosis, renal, 130

Vegetations, aortic valve, *223, 224*
Ventricular ectopics, 86, 244
　interpolated, *199, 200, 205, 206*
Ventricular fibrillation, 71
Ventricular septal defect, 88, 116, *211, 215*
Ventriculography, radionuclide, 87
Verapamil, 122

Warfarin, 54, 55, 235, 250
Wolff-Parkinson-White syndrome, 67, 121, *194, 204*

Zieve's syndrome, *199, 205*